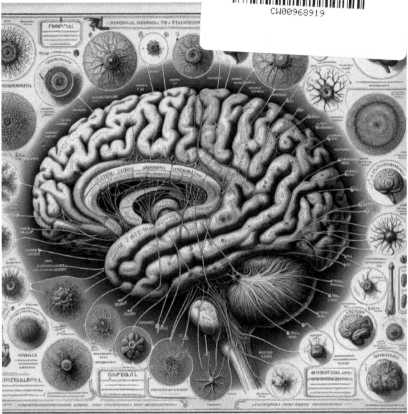

Understanding The Body The Brain

Understanding The Body, Volume 1

Robert Jakobsen

Published by Robert Jakobsen, 2024.

While every precaution has been taken in the preparation of this book, the publisher assumes no responsibility for errors or omissions, or for damages resulting from the use of the information contained herein.

UNDERSTANDING THE BODY THE BRAIN

First edition. October 21, 2024.

Copyright © 2024 Robert Jakobsen.

ISBN: 979-8227546937

Written by Robert Jakobsen.

Table of Contents

Introduction to The Brain

Understanding Our Most Vital Organ

The brain, our most vital organ, is an intricate masterpiece that governs every aspect of our existence. This remarkable organ not only enables us to think, feel, and remember but also regulates basic bodily functions such as breathing and heartbeat. Its influence permeates every facet of our lives, from the most complex cognitive processes to the simplest tasks we perform effortlessly. A mere three-pound mass concealed within the confines of our skull, the human brain towers above all else in its impact on our daily lives, behavior, and overall well-being. Understanding the brain's structure, function, and interconnected networks is like embarking on a captivating journey into the essence of what makes us uniquely human. It allows us to comprehend the marvels of human cognition and the intricate web of intricate processes that define our thoughts, emotions, and actions. As we delve deeper into this exploration, we find ourselves standing at the crossroads of countless awe-inspiring discoveries, each unveiling a new layer of complexity and wonder. Our understanding of the brain's inner workings empowers us to appreciate the profound implications it holds for our individual experiences and collective humanity. Through this lens of appreciation, we are drawn closer to the heart of our own existence, fueling our insatiable desire to unravel the mysteries of this extraordinary organ that shapes our very being.

The Wonder of Human Cognition

Human cognition is a wondrous phenomenon that has captivated the minds of thinkers, philosophers, and scientists for centuries. It encompasses the intricate processes of perception, attention, memory, language, problem-solving, and decision-making that define the essence of human intelligence. Each facet of cognition unveils an awe-inspiring blend of biological, psychological, and social influences that shape our thoughts, actions, and interactions with the world. From the remarkable ability to perceive and interpret sensory information to the intricacies of higher-order thinking, the complexities of human cognition continue to fascinate and perplex in equal measure. At the core of human cognition lies the enigmatic nature of consciousness, the subjective experience of being aware and engaged with the world. Our conscious experiences, ranging from mundane daily routines to profound moments of insight, reflect the vast landscape of cognitive processes that unfold within our minds. Whether we contemplate the enigma of creativity, grapple with the puzzles of logical reasoning, or marvel at the nuances of emotional perception, the realm of human cognition proves boundless in its intrigue and significance. It serves as the foundation upon which our understanding of ourselves, our relationships, and our place in the universe is built. Moreover, human cognition transcends individuality to embody a collective endeavor that shapes cultures, societies, and civilizations. It underpins the progression of knowledge, the development of technologies, and the evolution of belief systems, offering a testament to the power of the human mind to innovate, adapt, and create. The wonder of human cognition becomes palpable as we witness the myriad ways in which human thought combines with imagination and ingenuity to drive progress and transformation across diverse domains. From the realms of art and literature to the realms of science and philosophy, the influence of human cognition resounds through the annals of human history, leaving an indelible mark on the tapestry of human existence. As we delve into the depths of human cognition, we venture into a realm where the boundaries between the known and the unknown blur, inviting us to embrace the complexity, the mysteries, and the revelations that await. Exploring the wonder of human cognition offers a journey of introspection, discovery, and enlightenment that enriches our understanding of what it means to be human. It beckons us to ponder the infinite potential of the human mind and the unending quest to unravel the secrets woven within the fabric of cognition.

History of Brain Research

Throughout human history, our curiosity about the brain has been a driving force behind advancements in science and medicine. From the earliest observations of brain function by ancient scholars to the modern era of sophisticated neuroimaging techniques, the quest to understand the complexity of the brain has shaped our civilization's pursuit of knowledge. The history of brain research is a captivating narrative filled with breakthroughs, setbacks, and perseverance. Ancient civilizations, including the Egyptians and Greeks, recognized the brain as a vital organ, but their understanding was limited by the lack of scientific methods and technologies that we have today. It wasn't until the Renaissance period that significant progress was made in the study of the brain, with pioneering figures such as Leonardo da Vinci and Andreas Vesalius laying the foundations for modern neuroscience by conducting detailed anatomical studies. Advancements in technology further propelled the field forward, with the invention of the microscope opening new frontiers for investigating the intricate structures of the brain. The 19th and 20th centuries witnessed remarkable leaps in brain research, driven by scientists like Santiago Ramón y Cajal, who revolutionized our understanding of the nervous system through his discoveries of neuronal structure. The development of electroencephalography (EEG), computed tomography (CT), and magnetic resonance imaging (MRI) allowed researchers to delve deeper into the inner workings of the brain, unlocking mysteries that were once beyond our grasp. As we reflect on this historical journey, it becomes evident that each era has contributed to our present-day knowledge of the brain, paving the way for innovative treatments, interventions, and therapies that have improved countless lives. Acknowledging the rich tapestry of scientific inquiry that has brought us to where we are today, we are inspired to continue unraveling the enigma of the human brain, cherishing the legacy of those who laid the groundwork and embracing the possibilities that lie ahead.

Why the Brain Matters to You

The human brain, with its remarkable complexity and astonishing capabilities, is the very essence of our being. It is the command center for all our thoughts, emotions, behaviors, and bodily functions. Understanding the brain is not just a matter of scientific curiosity; it directly impacts every aspect of our lives. From the way we communicate and relate to others, to our ability to learn, adapt, and persevere in the face of challenges, the brain influences it all. At a fundamental level, the brain shapes our identity and defines who we are as individuals. Moreover, an awareness of brain health is crucial for maintaining overall well-being. The brain is susceptible to various disorders and illnesses that can have profound effects on our quality of life. Additionally, advancements in neuroscience continue to uncover groundbreaking insights into mental health, cognition, and consciousness, shedding light on the complexities of the human experience. By delving into the workings of the brain, you will gain a deeper appreciation for the marvels of the human mind and body. Ultimately, understanding the brain is empowering, as it equips us with knowledge that can enhance our physical and mental resilience, improve our relationships, and foster a greater sense of empathy and compassion. With this newfound insight, you will be better equipped to navigate the intricacies of your own thoughts and feelings, cultivate emotional intelligence, and promote holistic wellness. Therefore, the brain matters to you because it is the core of your existence, the key to your potential, and the gateway to a richer, more meaningful life.

How This Book Will Help

This book has been crafted with the utmost dedication and expertise to serve as your comprehensive guide to understanding the intricate workings of the human brain. Through this literary journey, we aim to unravel the complexities of the brain in a manner that is accessible, informative, and engaging. Our primary goal is to equip you with a profound insight into the marvels of the brain and empower you to make informed decisions pertaining to cognitive health and overall well-being. By delving deep into the realms of neuroscience, psychology, biology, and medicine, this book will foster a multidimensional understanding of the brain's functions, structure, and potential. Whether you are seeking to enhance your own cognitive abilities, support a loved one with cognitive challenges, or simply satisfy your intellectual curiosity, this book is poised to offer invaluable knowledge and practical guidance. Through a meticulous blend of scientific research, real-life anecdotes, and expert perspectives, you will gain a holistic perspective on the brain and its influence on every facet of human existence. Moreover, we have undertaken great care to present this information in a manner that is not only educational but also engrossing, ensuring that you are fully absorbed in the fascinating world of the brain throughout your reading journey. Additionally, as the field of neuroscience continues to evolve, this book will strive to keep you abreast of the latest advancements and breakthroughs. We are committed to delivering up-to-date insights and perspectives that reflect the dynamic nature of brain research, thereby empowering you to stay informed about the most recent developments in this rapidly advancing field. Furthermore, by offering practical strategies for nurturing cognitive wellness and advocating for the destigmatization of mental health, we aspire to cultivate a community of individuals who recognize the importance of prioritizing brain health and supporting those grappling with neurological conditions. It is our sincere hope that this book serves as a source of empathy, encouragement, and enlightenment for all who seek to enrich their understanding of the brain and its boundless capabilities.

Setting the Stage for Learning

In delving deeper into the intricate world of the brain, we embark on an enlightening journey that seeks to unravel the complexities of this remarkable organ. As we navigate through the intricacies of the human brain, we endeavor to create a foundation for learning that is both immersive and enriching. Understanding the brain's structure and functions can often be daunting, yet it is also deeply rewarding as it opens the door to a profound appreciation for the marvels of neuroscience. By setting the stage for learning, we lay the groundwork for a transformative experience that transcends mere information – it beckons us to comprehend the very essence of what makes us human. Every revelation about the brain unveils a new layer of understanding, shedding light on the intricate mechanisms that govern our thoughts, emotions, and behaviors. This chapter serves as a catalyst for intellectual exploration, fostering a genuine curiosity that inspires a lifelong dedication to unraveling the enigma of the human brain. Together, let us embrace the challenge of comprehending the brain's complexity, knowing that each insight gained brings us closer to appreciating the extraordinary tapestry of human cognition.

A Journey Through Complexity

The human brain is a magnificently complex organ that serves as the epicenter of our existence. Its intricacies and capabilities are awe-inspiring, encompassing numerous interconnected systems that govern everything from basic bodily functions to highly sophisticated cognitive processes. As we delve into the labyrinthine pathways of the brain, we begin to uncover the astonishing tapestry of neurons, synapses, and neurotransmitters that form the foundation of our thoughts, emotions, and behaviors. Every neural connection represents a mesmerizing feat of biological engineering, culminating in the wondrous symphony of consciousness. Navigating this terrain requires an appreciation of its boundless complexities. From the sensory cortex responsible for processing external stimuli to the prefrontal cortex governing executive functions, each region of the brain contributes to the holistic framework of human experience. We are propelled into a realm where the delicate balance of neurotransmitters bridges the realms of perception, memory, and learning. And amidst this complexity, we discover the brain's remarkable plasticity, allowing it to adapt and rewire itself in response to experiences and challenges. Yet, this journey through complexity extends beyond the confines of neurobiology. It leads us to ponder the intricate interplay between the physical and emotional aspects of our mental landscape. Our exploration unveils the impact of stress, trauma, and resilience on the brain, illustrating the profound implications for mental well-being. We are confronted with the enthralling enigma of creativity, as the brain weaves together disparate threads of inspiration, imagination, and ingenuity. Moreover, the unfolding narrative of brain development from infancy to old age invites us to contemplate the evolution of identity and wisdom. In traversing this terrain, we are humbled by the myriad ways in which the brain shapes our interactions with the world. Neuroplasticity reminds us of the potential for growth and healing, offering hope in the face of adversity. The complexities of mental health and neurological disorders beckon us to embrace empathy and understanding, advocating for destigmatization and compassionate support. Ultimately, this exploration unearths the fundamental truth that the journey through complexity is not merely an academic pursuit, but a profound odyssey that reflects the essence of our humanity.

Embracing Curiosity and Knowledge

In the exploration of the intricate landscape of the brain, one must wholeheartedly embrace curiosity and thirst for knowledge. This unfathomable organ, with its countless neurons forming complex pathways, invites us to delve into a realm where each discovery leads to even more profound questions. There is an inherent beauty in the pursuit of understanding the nuances of human cognition, and it is our sincere hope that this journey will ignite a fervent passion for learning within you. Embracing curiosity allows for the recognition of the sheer marvel encapsulated within the enigmatic folds of the brain, serving as an invitation to unravel the mysteries that have captivated the minds of scientists, philosophers, and scholars throughout centuries. Every turn of the page brings the opportunity to expand your knowledge, to challenge preconceived notions, and to revel in the wonder of the human intellect. It is through curiosity that new perspectives emerge, widening the horizon of our collective understanding. Beyond the allure of discovery, embracing knowledge entails a willingness to immerse oneself fully in the wealth of information presented. Equipped with a discerning mind and an open heart, one can absorb the intricacies of neuroscientific findings, appreciate the historical significance of landmark studies, and contemplate the implications of psychological theories. Each morsel of knowledge obtained creates a tapestry that threads together the fabric of our intellectual growth and fosters an appreciation for the incomparable complexities of our brains. By immersing ourselves in the pursuit of knowledge, we engage in a timeless dance with the profound ideas and insights that resonate across disciplines and generations. The very act of seeking knowledge serves as a testament to our innate desire to comprehend the inner workings of the brain and all its extraordinary capabilities. It is through this genuine embrace of curiosity and eagerness for knowledge that we embark on a transformational odyssey — one that promises to unlock the boundless potential of the mind while nurturing an unwavering respect for the mysteries that continue to both awe and inspire.

Key Concepts to Explore

As we delve deeper into the fascinating realm of brain science, it's essential to grasp key concepts that form the foundation of our understanding. One pivotal concept is neuroplasticity, the brain's remarkable ability to reorganize itself by forming new connections between neurons. This phenomenon underpins our capacity for learning, adaptation, and recovery from injury. Understanding neurotransmitters and their role in facilitating communication among brain cells is equally crucial. These chemical messengers play a vital role in regulating mood, memory, and various bodily functions, influencing our overall well-being. Another fundamental concept is the balance between the limbic system, responsible for our emotions, and the prefrontal cortex, governing rational thinking and decision-making. Recognizing this interplay can shed light on our behavior and reactions in different situations. Moreover, delving into the intricacies of synaptic pruning, where unnecessary connections are eliminated to enhance efficiency, offers profound insights into brain development and aging. Exploring the concept of cognitive reserve unveils the brain's ability to withstand neurological damage owing to its adaptive and resilient nature. Moreover, the concept of brain lateralization, delineating the functional asymmetry between the brain's left and right hemispheres, has significant implications for understanding individual differences in cognitive abilities and preferences. Furthermore, unraveling the delicate equilibrium between excitation and inhibition within the brain's neural networks provides valuable insights into various neurological disorders and their potential treatments. In addition, comprehending the principles of brain plasticity in response to environmental enrichment, mental stimulation, and physical exercise empowers us to harness these factors for optimal brain health and function. Lastly, examining the concept of epigenetics sheds light on how environmental factors and lifestyle choices can influence gene expression and subsequently impact brain health. By grasping these key concepts and their intricate interrelationships, we begin to appreciate the marvels of the brain and gain valuable insights into enhancing our cognitive well-being.

Our Commitment to Your Understanding

We are deeply committed to ensuring that you not only grasp the intricacies of the brain but also develop a profound appreciation for its remarkable capabilities. Throughout this book, our primary aim is to empower you with the knowledge and tools necessary to comprehend the complexities of the human brain. The journey we embark on together will delve into the depths of neuroscience, providing insights and understanding in a manner that is accessible and engaging. By fostering an environment of curiosity and exploration, we aspire to instill in you a sense of wonder and awe for the intricate workings of this miraculous organ. It is our earnest desire that every page you turn serves to illuminate and enlighten, unraveling the mysteries of the brain in a way that expands your cognitive horizons. As we proceed, know that our dedication to clarity and depth of understanding remains unwavering. We strive to offer explanations that are both informative and captivating, drawing you into the world of neuroscience and leaving you with a newfound admiration for the brain's astounding capabilities. By cultivating a deep understanding of the brain, we aim to equip you with the knowledge to make informed decisions about your health and well-being. Rest assured, our commitment to your understanding is unwavering, and we are wholeheartedly dedicated to guiding you through this enlightening journey of discovery.

Anatomy and Function

Understanding Brain Basics

The brain is an incredibly intricate and enigmatic organ, essential for sustaining life and orchestrating all bodily functions. Understanding its fundamental principles is crucial in comprehending our experiences, behaviors, and emotions. At the core of these basics lies the brain's remarkable structure, a marvel of nature that comprises different regions with specialized functions. From the cerebrum, which governs conscious thought and voluntary movement, to the cerebellum, responsible for coordination and balance, each macro structure plays a pivotal role in shaping our existence. The brainstem, often dubbed the body's autopilot, regulates essential processes such as breathing, heart rate, and sleep cycles. Delving into brain basics elucidates the intricate connections between these structures, highlighting the dazzling complexity that underpins human cognition. Moreover, studying the brain basics unveils its incredible adaptability – a quality known as neuroplasticity. This phenomenon enables the brain to rewire itself in response to new experiences, learning, and recovery from injury or trauma. As we further explore these aspects, we gain a profound appreciation for the brain's resilience and its capacity to evolve. Indeed, understanding brain basics goes beyond mere knowledge; it fosters awe and admiration for this marvel that defines our humanity.

Macro Structures of the Brain

The macro structures of the brain form the foundation of our cognitive and physiological functions, orchestrating a symphony of complex processes vital for our existence. At the helm sits the cerebrum, the largest part of the brain, responsible for higher-order thinking, sensory interpretation, and voluntary muscle movements. Beneath the cerebrum lies the cerebellum, often referred to as the 'little brain,' dedicated to precise coordination of motor movements, posture, and balance. Operating as the bridge between the spinal cord and the rest of the brain, the brainstem regulates fundamental bodily functions such as breathing, heartbeat, and consciousness, emphasizing its indispensable role in sustaining life. The intricate network of these macro structures not only supports our physical activities but also houses the neurological substrates for consciousness, emotion, and decision-making. As we delve into the intricacies of each region, we uncover the astonishing interplay that defines our human experience. Every structure, from the frontal lobe's executive functions to the parietal lobe's spatial awareness, contributes uniquely to our perception of the world. Moreover, the limbic system, comprising various brain regions, governs our emotional responses and memory consolidation, forming the core of our subjective experiences. Understanding the macro structures of the brain provides invaluable insights into the symbiotic relationship between our physical and mental well-being. By comprehending the roles played by these regions, we gain a profound appreciation for the remarkably orchestrated system that is the human brain, affirming its centrality in defining who we are as individuals.

Micro Anatomy: Neurons and Synapses

The micro anatomy of the brain is a fascinating subject that delves into the intricate details of neurons and synapses. Neurons are the fundamental building blocks of the nervous system, responsible for transmitting information through electrical and chemical signals. These cells form a complex network that enables the brain to process and respond to the various stimuli it encounters. Within each neuron, an elaborate system of dendrites, cell body, and axon work together to ensure the efficient transmission of signals. The synapses, which are the connections between neurons, play a crucial role in this communication process. They facilitate the transfer of information from one neuron to another, allowing for the seamless relay of messages throughout the brain. Understanding the micro anatomy of neurons and synapses provides insight into how the brain functions at a cellular level. It offers a glimpse into the incredible complexities underlying our thoughts, emotions, and behaviors. Moreover, exploring this topic sheds light on the mechanisms behind learning, memory formation, and various neurological conditions. Studying the micro anatomy of the brain fosters a deeper appreciation for the marvels of the human mind and the sophisticated machinery driving its operations. As we unravel the intricacies of neurons and synapses, we gain valuable knowledge that can ultimately inform advancements in neuroscience, medicine, and cognitive enhancement. This pursuit of understanding at the micro level opens doors to transformative discoveries that may revolutionize how we perceive and care for the most vital organ in the human body.

The Brain's Role in the Nervous System

The brain is a marvel of evolution, serving as the command center of the body's nervous system. It coordinates and controls an intricate network responsible for transmitting signals between different parts of the body. The nervous system can be categorized into two main divisions: the central nervous system (CNS) and the peripheral nervous system (PNS). The CNS, which consists of the brain and the spinal cord, is the core mechanism for processing and interpreting sensory information. On the other hand, the PNS extends throughout the body and connects the CNS to the limbs and organs. This extensive network of nerves enables the brain to communicate with every part of the body, regulating various physical and cognitive functions. Understanding the brain's role within this complex system sheds light on how it influences our day-to-day experiences. From the simplest reflex actions to the most elaborate thought processes, the brain orchestrates an astonishing array of functions. Furthermore, the brain's involvement in the autonomic nervous system ensures that crucial involuntary actions, such as heartbeat and breathing, are regulated seamlessly, reflecting the remarkable efficiency of this biological supercomputer. Appreciating the brain's pivotal role in maintaining homeostasis and coordinating responses to internal and external stimuli deepens our admiration for the intricacies of the human body. The complexity and interconnectedness of the brain and the nervous system contribute to the awe-inspiring nature of the human experience, serving as a testament to the marvels of nature.

Regions and Their Functions

The human brain, with its awe-inspiring complexity, is a marvel of natural engineering. It is composed of various regions, each with distinct functions crucial to our daily lives. The cerebral cortex, the outermost layer of the brain, can be divided into four main lobes: frontal, parietal, temporal, and occipital. Each lobe boasts its own specialized responsibilities. The frontal lobe, positioned at the front of the brain, is involved in decision-making, problem-solving, and emotions. Meanwhile, the parietal lobe deals with sensory information and spatial awareness, assisting us in comprehending our surroundings and coordinating our movements. The temporal lobe contributes to memory, language, and auditory processing, fostering our ability to recognize sounds and comprehend speech. Lastly, the occipital lobe, nestled at the back of the brain, is dedicated to visual processing, enabling the interpretation of what we see. Beyond these lobes, deeper structures such as the thalamus and hypothalamus play integral roles in relaying sensory and motor signals, regulating sleep, thirst, hunger, and other primal instincts. Equally significant are the cerebellum and brainstem, which govern coordination and automatic functions like breathing and heart rate. With this intricate web of specialized areas, the human brain orchestrates the symphony of our thoughts, actions, and emotions. Understanding these regions and their intricate functions is key to appreciating the unique capabilities of the human mind.

Communication Pathways

The brain is a marvel of communication, with its various regions and systems working in harmony to facilitate internal and external interactions. Communication pathways within the brain are crucial for transmitting information, coordinating responses, and maintaining overall cognitive function. At the core of these complex pathways are the intricate networks of neurons and synapses, which form the basis for all communication within the brain. These networks enable the transmission of electrical signals, allowing for rapid and precise communication between different regions of the brain. Furthermore, these pathways play a fundamental role in integrating sensory input, motor output, and higher-order cognitive processes. Through these pathways, the brain is able to process and interpret a vast array of stimuli from the environment, and coordinate appropriate behavioral and physiological responses. The communication pathways also serve as the foundation for vital functions such as language processing, decision-making, and emotional regulation. It's fascinating to consider how these pathways facilitate the seamless exchange of information that underpins our thoughts, actions, and experiences. Moreover, disturbances in these pathways can lead to various neurological and psychiatric conditions, highlighting their significance in maintaining overall brain health. Understanding the organization and functionality of these communication pathways is thus essential for gaining insights into brain disorders and developing effective interventions. As we delve deeper into the intricate web of communication pathways, we uncover the remarkable complexity and resilience of the human brain, shedding light on the extraordinary mechanisms that drive our cognitive and emotional lives.

Sensory Processing Essentials

Our brain's ability to process and interpret sensory information is fundamental to our day-to-day experiences. Sensory processing encompasses the way our nervous system receives, organizes, and interprets stimuli from the environment. It involves a remarkable orchestration of various sensory modalities, including touch, taste, smell, sight, and hearing, to create a unified perception of the world around us. Within the intricate neural networks of the brain, dedicated regions are responsible for processing specific sensory inputs. The thalamus serves as the central relay station, directing sensory information to the appropriate cortical areas for further processing and interpretation. Each sensory modality follows distinct pathways, converging and interacting within the cortex to construct our rich sensory experiences. Furthermore, sensory processing extends beyond mere detection of stimuli. It involves perceptual organization, where the brain integrates multiple sensory cues to form a cohesive understanding of our environment. For instance, the brain effortlessly combines sound and visual input to create a seamless perception of a bustling city street or a tranquil countryside. Notably, sensory processing is not uniform across individuals. Variations in sensory sensitivity and perception can significantly impact how we experience the world. Conditions like autism spectrum disorders or sensory processing disorders underscore the diverse ways in which our brains receive and interpret sensory information, highlighting the extraordinary complexity of sensory processing. Understanding the nuances of sensory processing is crucial in various aspects of life, from optimizing learning environments for children to creating accessible spaces for individuals with sensory sensitivities. Moreover, appreciating the intricacies of sensory processing fosters empathy and understanding, enabling us to better support those with unique sensory experiences. In essence, delving into the essentials of sensory processing unveils the remarkable capabilities of the human brain, shaping our perceptions, interactions, and overall experiences. By unraveling the mysteries of sensory processing, we gain profound insights into what makes each individual's encounter with the world truly unique and awe-inspiring.

Language and Cognition Functions

Language and cognition are fundamental aspects of human existence, and the brain plays a central role in both. The intricate dance between language and cognition is a captivating area of study that continues to reveal the astonishing capacities of the human mind. As we explore the brain's remarkable ability to process language and facilitate higher cognitive functions, we gain invaluable insights into what makes us uniquely human. The brain's language functions encompass an astonishing array of processes, from understanding speech to formulating complex sentences and expressing thoughts and emotions. Broca's area, located in the frontal lobe, is known for its involvement in speech production and articulation, while Wernicke's area, situated in the temporal lobe, is essential for language comprehension. These interconnected regions work harmoniously to enable the seamless expression and comprehension of language, highlighting the remarkable efficiency of the brain's linguistic capabilities. Cognition, on the other hand, involves the complex mental processes that enable us to acquire knowledge, comprehend ideas, solve problems, and make decisions. Executive functions, such as attention, memory, and problem-solving, rely on the coordinated efforts of various brain regions, including the prefrontal cortex and the hippocampus. These areas play crucial roles in orchestrating our cognitive abilities, allowing us to navigate the complexities of daily life with grace and acumen. Moreover, the intricate interplay between language and cognition is evident in the way we use language to shape our thoughts and convey our innermost feelings. Words serve as vessels for our ideas, emotions, and experiences, allowing us to share our worldviews and connect with others on a profound level. This symbiotic relationship illuminates the profound influence of language on our cognitive processes, underscoring the profound impact of linguistic fluency on our mental agility and creativity. In the realm of neuroscientific research, ongoing investigations continue to unveil the mysteries of language and cognition, shedding light on the neural underpinnings of bilingualism, language acquisition, and the impact of communication disorders on cognitive function. Each discovery deepens our appreciation for the intricacies of the brain's linguistic and cognitive machinery, unveiling the extraordinary depth and resilience of our mental faculties. As we deepen our understanding of the brain's language and cognition functions, we embark on a riveting journey into the essence of human consciousness. The enduring allure of this field lies in its capacity to unravel the enigma of human thought and expression, offering profound insights into the nature of our minds and the infinite potential they possess.

Memory and Learning Mechanisms

Memory and learning are fundamental aspects of human cognition, shaping our experiences, behaviors, and overall understanding of the world. The intricate mechanisms behind memory formation and retention provide a profound insight into the capabilities of the human brain. When we experience something new, our brains undergo a complex process to encode and store this information. This process involves various regions of the brain working in harmony, including the hippocampus, amygdala, and prefrontal cortex. Memories are not stored in a single location in the brain; rather, they are distributed across different regions, each playing a specific role in the retrieval and association of memories. Additionally, our ability to learn is closely intertwined with memory processes. Learning occurs through the acquisition of new knowledge or skills, while memory enables us to retain and utilize the acquired information in the future. Understanding the neural mechanisms of memory formation and learning has significant implications in education, psychology, and neuroscience. For instance, studying the impact of various factors on memory formation, such as emotions, repetition, and associations, sheds light on effective learning strategies and educational practices. Moreover, examining the differences in memory and learning abilities across individuals provides valuable insights into cognitive development and potential interventions for memory-related conditions. Neuroplasticity, the brain's remarkable ability to reorganize and adapt, plays a crucial role in memory and learning. It allows the brain to form new neural connections, strengthen existing ones, and reconfigure its networks in response to experiences and learning processes. This phenomenon underlies the concept of lifelong learning and highlights the brain's capacity for continual growth and development throughout an individual's life. Furthermore, exploring the influence of external factors, such as stress, sleep, and nutrition, on memory and learning elucidates the holistic nature of cognitive processes. Optimal mental and physical well-being supports enhanced memory performance and efficient learning, emphasizing the interconnectedness of various aspects of human health with cognitive functions. In summary, delving into memory and learning mechanisms not only unveils the marvels of the human brain but also offers practical implications for enhancing educational practices, understanding cognitive development, and addressing cognitive challenges. By appreciating the complexities and intricacies of memory and learning, we gain deeper insights into the capabilities of our remarkable brains and pave the way for continuous intellectual enrichment and cognitive well-being.

Balancing Act: Emotions and Homeostasis

Understanding the complex interplay between emotions and homeostasis is crucial in deciphering the intricate workings of the brain. Emotions, often thought of as abstract feelings, actually stem from a finely tuned regulation of various neurochemicals and neural pathways. These mechanisms are essential for maintaining a state of equilibrium within the body, known as homeostasis. The brain's limbic system, comprising the amygdala, hippocampus, and hypothalamus, plays a central role in orchestrating emotional responses and regulating physiological balance. When we experience emotional stimuli, such as fear, joy, or sadness, these regions are activated, triggering a cascade of hormonal and neuronal signals that influence our bodily functions. For instance, the fight-or-flight response elicited by the amygdala can rapidly elevate heart rate and increase stress hormone levels in preparation for a perceived threat. Conversely, feelings of contentment or love may lead to the release of oxytocin, promoting relaxation and bonding. Additionally, the intricate connection between emotions and homeostasis extends to behaviors such as eating, drinking, and sleeping. Emotional cues can significantly impact our appetite, hydration levels, and sleep patterns, all of which are vital components of physiological balance. Disruptions in this delicate interplay can manifest as mood disorders, anxiety, or even physical ailments. Understanding how emotions and homeostasis are intertwined sheds light on the profound impact of mental well-being on overall health. By delving into the intricate dance between neural circuitry, hormones, and behavior, we gain insight into the holistic nature of emotional regulation and its fundamental importance in maintaining a harmonious internal environment.

The Role of Vitamins and Nutrients

A Heartfelt Introduction to Nutrients

In delving into the fascinating world of mental health, we come to realize the profound significance of nutrients in nourishing and sustaining not just our bodies, but also our minds. The intricate relationship between nutrition and mental well-being has captivated researchers and health enthusiasts alike for decades. It is a testament to the pivotal role that essential vitamins and nutrients play in shaping our cognitive functions, emotional stability, and overall mental resilience. As we embark on this journey of exploration, it becomes increasingly evident that the vitamins and nutrients we consume are not merely elements to fill our stomachs, but rather crucial components that directly impact our psychological vitality. The revelation of this connection serves as a poignant reminder of the intertwined nature of physical and mental health. Our quest to unravel the mysteries of mental well-being must encompass a holistic approach that celebrates the nurturing power of nutrients. Through this profound understanding, we strive to honor the genuine essence of nourishment, recognizing its ability to fortify, replenish, and uplift our cognitive and emotional capacities. It is with an earnest heart that we delve deeper into the realm of nutrients, acknowledging their unwavering influence in fostering a resilient and flourishing mind.

The Building Blocks: Essential Vitamins Explained

Vitamins are the essential building blocks that support our overall health and well-being. They play a crucial role in various bodily functions, from supporting the immune system to aiding in proper growth and development. Each vitamin brings its own unique benefits, contributing to the intricate balance of our biological systems. Vitamin A, for instance, is renowned for promoting good vision, healthy skin, and a robust immune system. It acts as a powerful antioxidant, protecting cells from damage caused by free radicals. Moving on to

Vitamin B complex, these water-soluble vitamins are crucial for turning food into energy and maintaining a healthy metabolism. They also support the nervous system and aid in the production of red blood cells. Vitamin C, another vital nutrient, is celebrated for its immune-boosting properties and ability to promote collagen production, essential for skin elasticity and wound healing. Meanwhile, Vitamin D is instrumental in maintaining strong bones and teeth, as it helps the body absorb calcium. Furthermore, it plays a role in supporting immune function and regulating mood. Lastly, Vitamin E, known for its antioxidant properties, helps protect cells from damage and supports immune function. Understanding the role of each essential vitamin empowers us to make informed decisions about our diet and lifestyle choices as we strive to prioritize our health. It is paramount to ensure an adequate intake of these vital nutrients through a balanced and varied diet, underlining the significance of incorporating a wide array of fruits, vegetables, lean proteins, and whole grains into our daily meals. By embracing the value of essential vitamins and their profound impact on our well-being, we take a significant step towards nurturing our bodies and minds.

Minerals: The Unsung Heroes of Wellness

Minerals are the unsung heroes of wellness, quietly but tirelessly supporting various bodily functions essential to our well-being. From calcium for strong bones and teeth to iron for oxygen transportation in the blood, minerals play a pivotal role in maintaining our health. Often overshadowed by the spotlight on vitamins, these micronutrients deserve much more recognition for their contributions to overall wellness. One key mineral that merits attention is magnesium, known for its multifaceted roles in the body. Magnesium is involved in over 300 enzymatic reactions, including energy production and nerve function, making it crucial for maintaining vitality and cognitive sharpness. Its calming effect on the nervous system also promotes relaxation and quality sleep, vital components of holistic well-being.

Selenium, another unsung hero, acts as a powerful antioxidant, protecting cells from oxidative damage and bolstering the immune system. This trace mineral is essential for thyroid function and proper DNA synthesis, emphasizing its significance in maintaining overall health and vibrant vitality. Additionally, zinc, although often overlooked, plays a critical role in immune function, wound healing, and maintaining the senses of taste and smell. Moving beyond the physical impact, minerals also contribute significantly to mental and emotional wellness. For instance, the role of copper in brain function highlights its importance beyond its well-known use in electrical wiring and plumbing. Copper supports the production of neurotransmitters and assists in forming the myelin sheath that insulates nerve fibers, thereby contributing to optimal nervous system function. In today's constantly evolving wellness landscape, the appreciation for minerals is gaining momentum as their significance becomes increasingly recognized. It is imperative that we acknowledge and emphasize the integral role they play in achieving and maintaining good health. As we strive for comprehensive well-being, nurturing our bodies with a diverse array of minerals is paramount. Let us shine a brighter light on these unsung heroes and embrace the profound impact they have on our overall wellness.

Omega-3 and the Brain's Lifeline

Omega-3 fatty acids have long been revered for their remarkable impact on brain health and overall well-being. These essential fats, which include EPA (eicosapentaenoic acid) and DHA (docosahexaenoic acid), play a pivotal role in supporting cognitive function, emotional stability, and neurological development. Research has consistently shown that omega-3s are crucial components of the brain's cellular membranes, influencing signal transmission and synaptic plasticity. Furthermore, these nutrients have been linked to reducing inflammation in the brain, which is associated with various neurological disorders. In addition to their structural significance, omega-3 fatty acids also exert profound effects on neurotransmitter function. They are instrumental in regulating the release and uptake of key neurotransmitters such as serotonin and dopamine, which are integral to mood regulation and mental clarity. Notably, adequate levels of omega-3s have been associated with a reduced risk of depression and anxiety, highlighting their role in maintaining emotional equilibrium. Beyond mental health, omega-3s demonstrate an array of benefits for the entire body. Their anti-inflammatory properties extend to the cardiovascular system, where they promote healthy blood circulation and help maintain optimal blood pressure. Research suggests that omega-3 fatty acids may also contribute to reducing the risk of heart disease by improving lipid profiles and protecting against arterial plaque buildup. Moreover, the impact of omega-3s extends across the lifespan, from prenatal development to aging. During pregnancy, these essential nutrients are critical for fetal brain growth and development, and their consumption has been associated with improved cognitive outcomes in children. In later life, omega-3s continue to support cognitive function and may even play a role in preserving memory and cognitive agility. Given the essential nature of omega-3 fatty acids, it is crucial to incorporate dietary sources of these nutrients into our daily regimen. Fatty fish, such as salmon, mackerel, and sardines, are rich sources of EPA and DHA, making them invaluable additions to a brain-healthy diet. For individuals who prefer plant-based options, flaxseeds, chia seeds, and walnuts provide alpha-linolenic acid (ALA), a precursor to EPA and DHA. In recognition of their far-reaching benefits, omega-3s stand as a testament to the vital role that nutrition plays in nurturing the brain's resilience and vitality.

B-Vitamins: Energizing and Empowering

Our journey through the intricate world of nutrition brings us to a pivotal player in the realm of vitality and well-being – B-vitamins. These essential nutrients are revered for their unparalleled ability to invigorate and empower not only the body but also the mind. From bolstering energy levels to fortifying the nervous system, B-vitamins play an indispensable role in our overall health. Comprising a family of eight distinct members, including B1 (thiamine), B2 (riboflavin), B3 (niacin), B5 (pantothenic acid), B6 (pyridoxine), B7 (biotin), B9 (folate), and B12 (cobalamin), each member contributes uniquely to the symphony of bodily functions. At the core of their impact lies their ability to convert food into fuel, providing the vital energy needed for every cell and organ to thrive. As we delve deeper into the unique attributes of each B-vitamin, we uncover their significant roles in metabolism, cognitive function, and neurotransmitter synthesis. Furthermore, their influence in promoting red blood cell production and maintaining a healthy cardiovascular system cannot be overstated. This enlightening exploration will unveil how these mighty B-vitamins act as catalysts for countless biochemical reactions within the body, playing a paramount role in sustaining optimal health. Our sincere endeavor is to unravel the extensive benefits of B-vitamins, offering an insightful understanding that empowers individuals to make informed choices that nurture their well-being. Stay tuned as we embark on this enlightening odyssey to discover the inherent potency of B-vitamins in energizing and fortifying mind, body, and soul.

Antioxidants: Defenders Against Time

As we journey through the landscape of wellness, it's imperative to acknowledge the pivotal role that antioxidants play in preserving our vitality and defending against the relentless march of time. Antioxidants are the unsung champions that combat the damaging effects of free radicals, those unruly molecules that wreak havoc on our cells and accelerate the aging process. By neutralizing these free radicals, antioxidants safeguard our cells and contribute to overall health and well-being. Among the plethora of antioxidants, vitamin C stands out as a powerhouse defender. Renowned for its immune-boosting properties, vitamin C also aids in the repair and regeneration of tissues, reinforcing the body's resilience against external stressors. Additionally, the formidable duo of vitamins A and E work in harmony to shield the body from oxidative stress, guarding against cellular damage and bolstering skin health. Furthermore, the vibrant spectrum of plant-based antioxidants, including flavonoids and carotenoids, offers a diverse array of protective benefits. These natural compounds, found abundantly in fruits, vegetables, and legumes, act as nature's armor, fortifying the body against the corrosive impact of environmental pollutants and toxins. In embracing the profound impact of antioxidants, we unlock the potential to not only extend our longevity but also enhance the quality of our lives. By nurturing ourselves with antioxidant-rich foods and supplements, we actively engage in an enduring partnership with our bodies, fostering resilience, vitality, and a renewed sense of well-being. As we deepen our understanding of these mighty defenders, we open the door to a future characterized by strengthened immunity, heightened energy, and the graceful embrace of advancing years.

Balancing Act: Vitamins A, C, D & E

Vitamins A, C, D, and E play essential roles in sustaining our physical and mental well-being. Vitamin A, primarily found in colorful fruits and vegetables, is vital for maintaining healthy vision, promoting a robust immune system, and supporting cellular growth and function. Likewise, Vitamin C serves as a powerful antioxidant, aiding in the body's natural defense against harmful free radicals, while also contributing to the synthesis of collagen, which is crucial for skin health and wound healing. With its ability to enhance iron absorption and fortify the immune system, Vitamin C emerges as an indispensable ally in our pursuit of holistic wellness. Moving on to Vitamin D, often referred to as the 'sunshine vitamin', this nutrient plays a pivotal role in facilitating strong bones and teeth, regulating calcium levels, and bolstering immune function. Notably, it also holds promise in influencing mood and warding off depression, shedding light on its significance in nurturing both physical and emotional health. Lastly, Vitamin E, recognized for its potent antioxidant properties, supports skin health and inhibits oxidative stress, thereby safeguarding cells from damage. Its interaction with vitamins A and C further underscores the interconnectedness of these nutrients in fortifying our overall well-being. Achieving a harmonious balance of vitamins A, C, D, and E demands mindfulness in our dietary choices, incorporating a spectrum of natural sources such as leafy greens, citrus fruits, nuts, seeds, and fortified dairy products. This concerted effort not only fortifies our bodies with the necessary nourishment but also cultivates a deeper appreciation for the inherent beauty and resilience of nature's offerings. As we endeavor to leverage the combined potency of these vitamins, let us embrace the profound impact they wield in safeguarding our vitality and embracing a fulfilling, flourishing existence.

Nutrients that Nurture Mental Health

Mental health is a complex and multifaceted aspect of our overall well-being, intricately linked to the nutrients we consume. The pursuit of mental wellness encompasses more than just the absence of illness; it embodies a state of equilibrium, resilience, and emotional harmony that enables us to lead fulfilling lives. In this chapter, we will explore the profound impact that specific nutrients have on nurturing and sustaining mental health. Omega-3 fatty acids, particularly eicosapentaenoic acid (EPA) and docosahexaenoic acid (DHA), play an indispensable role in promoting optimal brain function and emotional stability. These essential fatty acids are vital components of cell membranes in the brain and are believed to influence neurotransmitter pathways, contributing to cognitive clarity and mood regulation. Incorporating sources of omega-3, such as oily fish, flaxseeds, and walnuts into our diets can aid in fortifying our mental resilience and combating conditions like anxiety and depression. Another essential nutrient linked to mental well-being is magnesium. This mineral is involved in hundreds of biochemical reactions within the body, including those related to neurotransmitter activity and stress response. Deficiencies in magnesium have been associated with heightened stress levels and an increased susceptibility to mood disorders. By embracing magnesium-rich foods like spinach, pumpkin seeds, and almonds, individuals can help support their mental equilibrium, fostering a sense of calm and emotional robustness. Furthermore, the role of B-vitamins, notably folate, vitamin B6, and vitamin B12, cannot be overstated in the realm of mental health. These vitamins are integral for the synthesis of neurotransmitters such as serotonin and dopamine, which are pivotal in regulating mood and emotional well-being. Insufficient levels of B-vitamins have been correlated with an elevated risk of depression and cognitive impairment. Introducing B-vitamin rich foods like leafy greens, legumes, and lean proteins into our diets can contribute to nurturing a positive mindset and enhancing cognitive acuity. In addition to these nutrients, the influence of antioxidants, particularly vitamin C and E, in safeguarding mental health should not be overlooked. Antioxidants play a crucial role in defending our brain cells from oxidative stress and inflammation, mechanisms implicated in the pathophysiology of mental disorders. By embracing a diet abundant in vibrant fruits, vegetables, and nuts, individuals can harness the protective prowess of antioxidants, reinforcing their mental resilience and cognitive vitality. As our understanding of the intricate interplay between nutrition and mental well-being deepens, it becomes increasingly evident that the foods we consume can profoundly shape our emotional equilibrium and cognitive fortitude. Nurturing our mental health through mindful, nutrient-dense dietary choices empowers us to cultivate inner strength, resilience, and emotional vitality, ultimately enriching our lived experiences.

Holistic View: Integrating Nutrition into Daily Life

Nutrition is not just about the food we eat—it's about nourishing our bodies, minds, and spirits. As we navigate the complexities of modern life, integrating nutrition into our daily routines becomes an essential aspect of overall wellbeing. It's about adopting a holistic view that recognizes the interconnectedness of our physical and mental health with the foods we consume. This section will explore practical ways to integrate nutrition into daily life, emphasizing the sincere importance of making mindful choices. Creating a Holistic Approach: Integrating nutrition into daily life involves more than just planning meals; it entails cultivating a mindset that values the impact of food on our overall wellness. This approach encourages individuals to consider the nutritional value of their meals, understand the source and quality of their food, and appreciate the journey from farm to table. By acknowledging the interconnectedness of our food choices with our health, we elevate the act of eating into a nourishing ritual. Mindful Eating Practices: The act of eating mindfully is fundamental to integrating nutrition into daily life. This involves savoring each bite, being present at meal times, and appreciating the sensory experience of eating. By cultivating mindful eating habits, individuals can develop a deep appreciation for the nourishment provided by each meal, leading to a healthier relationship with food. Additionally, being mindful of portion sizes and avoiding distractions during meals can greatly impact our overall satisfaction and fulfillment from eating. Meal Planning Made Sincere: Integrating nutrition into daily life necessitates thoughtful meal planning. By conscientiously selecting a variety of nutrient-dense foods, individuals can ensure they receive a spectrum of essential vitamins, minerals, and other vital nutrients. This approach also allows for the inclusion of diverse flavors and cuisines, adding an element of enjoyment to the practice of nourishing oneself. Creating a sincere space for meal preparation and sharing meals with loved ones can enhance the overall experience and foster a deeper connection to the value of good nutrition. Balancing Convenience and Nutritional Value: In our fast-paced world, convenience often takes precedence over nutritional value when it comes to food choices. However, integrating nutrition into daily life calls for a recalibration of these priorities. It involves seeking a balance between convenience and the nourishing properties of food. One can strive to incorporate quick, wholesome options without compromising the nutritional content. This could involve stocking up on nutritious snacks, preparing grab-and-go meals in advance, and choosing minimally processed, whole food options when time is of the essence. Cultivating Awareness and Gratitude: Integrating nutrition into daily life fosters a culture of awareness and gratitude. Becoming attuned to the benefits of consuming wholesome, nutrient-rich foods cultivates a sense of gratitude for the nourishment it provides. Embracing this perspective invites a shift in mindset—one that acknowledges the transformative power of nutrition in shaping our physical and emotional well-being. By fostering a conscious appreciation for the sustenance we receive, we infuse every meal with a sincere acknowledgment of its significance in supporting our vitality. In summary, integrating nutrition into daily life transcends the mere act of eating; it embodies a mindful, holistic, and sincere approach to nourishing our bodies and nurturing our well-being. By understanding the interplay between nutrition and daily living, individuals can embark on a journey toward a more balanced and fulfilling relationship with food.

A Sincere Reflection on Nourishing the Mind

As we reflect on the intricate relationship between nutrition and mental health, it becomes apparent that nourishing the mind is as crucial as nourishing the body. The concept of holistic well-being extends beyond physical sustenance to encompass emotional and psychological nourishment. When we speak of nurturing the mind, we delve into the profound impact of food and nutrients on cognitive function, emotional resilience, and overall mental wellness. Nourishing the mind transcends the mere act of consuming nutrients; it involves a mindful and conscientious approach to fueling the brain for optimal performance and emotional equilibrium. It's about recognizing the power of food not just to satiate hunger but also to stimulate clarity of thought, emotional balance, and sustained vitality. It's about fostering an intimate understanding of how various nutrients directly influence brain chemistry and functioning. When we sincerely reflect on nourishing the mind, we acknowledge the remarkable potential of certain foods and nutrients to support cognitive clarity, emotional stability, and long-term mental resilience. This reflection prompts us to appreciate the significance of a well-balanced diet rich in essential vitamins, minerals, and antioxidants. We come to understand the pivotal role that omega-3 fatty acids, B-vitamins, and other vital nutrients play in promoting mental acuity, emotional well-being, and even safeguarding against neurological decline. Furthermore, this reflection invites us to embrace a mindful and deliberate approach to our dietary choices, recognizing that what we consume not only fuels our bodies but also shapes our mental and emotional states. It encourages us to view food as a source of nourishment for both body and soul, advocating for a harmonious integration of nutritious eating habits and mindfulness practices. Through this reflection, we cultivate a deep sense of reverence for the profound connection between nourishment and mental wellness, fostering an enduring commitment to prioritize the health of our minds with the same sincerity as we do for our bodies.

Exercise and Physical Activity

Understanding Exercise: Beyond Just Movement

Exercise is often viewed simply as physical activity or movement designed to maintain or improve physical fitness, but it encompasses much more. When we engage in exercise, we are not just moving our bodies; we are also nurturing our minds and souls. Here, the mind-body connection becomes evident as exercise becomes an integral part of holistic health. The act of exercising taps into a deeper level of our being, fostering harmony between our mental and physical well-being. It's not just about lifting weights or running miles. It's about feeling the energy resonating through every cell in our body, invigorating and rejuvenating us from within. The impact of exercise ripples through our entire existence, bringing balance and vitality to our lives. By understanding exercise in this light, we can appreciate its transformative power. Through exercise, we learn to honor and respect our bodies. We become more attuned to our strengths and limitations while cultivating a profound sense of gratitude for what our bodies can achieve. Every step, every stretch, and every breath becomes a conscious and deliberate act of self-care. As we tread this path, we discover that exercise is not just a regimen but a sacred ritual that nourishes our whole being. It empowers us to overcome physical and mental barriers, teaching us resilience and determination. Most importantly, it provides us with moments of tranquility and peace amidst life's chaos. This understanding of exercise opens doors to endless possibilities for growth and transformation. It offers an opportunity for self-discovery and introspection, allowing us to explore untapped potential and unlock hidden strengths. As we delve deeper into the meaning of exercise, we realize that it is a holistic practice that embodies the essence of living fully. It's not a mere chore on our to-do list but a profound expression of gratitude, love, and devotion to ourselves. With each session, our bodies become more than vessels for movement; they become instruments of compassion and self-realization. Ultimately, exercise transcends the physical realm and becomes a journey towards self-fulfillment and well-being.

Connecting Body and Mind Through Activity

Physical activity is not just about the body; it is also deeply connected to the mind and spirit. Engaging in exercise creates a powerful avenue for mental and emotional well-being. The benefits of exercise extend beyond physical fitness and are often instrumental in shaping a positive outlook on life. When you partake in physical activities, your body releases chemicals called endorphins that trigger a positive feeling in the body. This rush of endorphins is often referred to as a 'runner's high,' and it can induce feelings of euphoria and minimize the perception of pain. Moreover, regular exercise has been shown to reduce stress, anxiety, and depression by enhancing the brain's ability to manage emotional states. It offers a natural way to improve mood and cope with daily challenges. Furthermore, physical activity strengthens the mind-body connection, allowing individuals to develop a deeper understanding and appreciation of their bodies. Whether it's through yoga, meditation, or simply going for a walk, exercising mindfulness during physical activity promotes a sense of harmony between the body and mind. As you engage in these activities, you become more attuned to the present moment, fostering a profound connection between your physical movements and mental awareness. This symbiotic relationship contributes to a more holistic and integrated sense of well-being. By deliberately bringing awareness to the sensations, movements, and breath during exercise, you can cultivate a deeper mind-body connection that enriches your overall experience. Additionally, embracing this interconnectedness can lead to increased self-awareness and a heightened ability to respond to the needs of both your body and mind. As you continue your journey of exploring different forms of physical activity, remember that the connection between your physical and mental health is an ongoing and transformative process. By nurturing this connection, you will gain a deeper appreciation for the profound impact that exercise has on both your body and mind.

Different Types of Exercises and Their Impact

Physical activity is not just about breaking a sweat or burning calories; it's about fostering a deeper connection between mind, body, and soul. When considering different types of exercises, it's crucial to understand their unique impacts on overall well-being. From the invigorating rush of cardiovascular workouts to the serene mindfulness of yoga and the empowering strength training sessions, each form of exercise offers distinct benefits. Cardio exercises, such as running, swimming, or cycling, elevate the heart rate, improve circulation, and boost endurance, leading to enhanced cardiovascular health. On the other hand, yoga promotes flexibility, balance, and mental tranquility, allowing for a harmonious alignment of physical and mental wellness. Strength training, whether through weightlifting or bodyweight exercises, builds muscle mass, strengthens bones, and bolsters confidence in one's physical capabilities. Furthermore, engaging in activities like dancing, hiking, or martial arts not only adds variety and excitement to one's fitness routine but also cultivates creativity, perseverance, and camaraderie. Understanding the impact of these diverse exercises empowers individuals to craft a holistic approach to their fitness journey, ensuring a balanced and fulfilling pursuit of well-being.

Listening to Your Body's Signals

As you engage in physical activity, it's crucial to tune into the cues that your body is sending you. Paying attention to these signals can make a profound difference in your overall well-being. Your body has an innate wisdom that communicates through various sensations and responses. It's essential to be mindful of these messages and be proactive in addressing them. One of the key aspects of listening to your body's signals is acknowledging discomfort versus pain. Discomfort might arise during exercise as a natural response to exertion, but it's important to differentiate it from true physical pain, which could signal potential injury or strain. By learning to recognize the nuances of these sensations, you can prevent unnecessary harm and optimize your workouts. Furthermore, observing your energy levels and fatigue patterns can provide valuable insights into your body's needs. Are you feeling invigorated and energized after a particular type of exercise, or are you experiencing persistent fatigue? These indicators can guide you in tailoring your fitness regimen to better suit your unique requirements. Additionally, being attuned to your body's signals involves understanding the impact of stress on your physical state. Stress manifests not only mentally but also physically, affecting muscle tension, posture, and breathing patterns. By honing in on these bodily responses, you can implement targeted relaxation techniques and lifestyle adjustments to mitigate the detrimental effects of stress. This heightened awareness can lead to a more harmonious connection between mind and body, fostering a holistic approach to health and fitness. Ultimately, by listening to your body's signals, you'll embark on a journey of self-discovery and self-care, nurturing a profound understanding of your physical and mental needs.

The Science Behind Endorphins

When we engage in physical activity, our bodies undergo a fantastic transformation. One of the most remarkable aspects of this change is the release of endorphins, often referred to as 'feel-good' hormones. These neurotransmitters are produced by the central nervous system and the pituitary gland in response to stress or pain. Their incredible ability to act as natural painkillers and mood elevators make them a fascinating subject of scientific study. Endorphins work their magic by binding to the opiate receptors in our brains, reducing our perception of pain and triggering feelings of euphoria. This chemical process not only diminishes discomfort during exercise, but also contributes to the much-celebrated 'runner's high' experienced by many athletes and fitness enthusiasts. Beyond the immediate post-workout glow, regular physical activity has been linked to long-term boosts in overall well-being and mental health, thanks in part to the consistent release of endorphins. In addition to their pain-relieving and mood-enhancing effects, endorphins play a crucial role in regulating appetite, releasing sex hormones, and enhancing the immune response. This multifaceted impact underscores the profound interconnectedness of physical activity and our body's biochemical processes. Understanding the science behind endorphins can empower individuals to harness the potential of these natural chemicals for their holistic health and wellness. It's important to note that the release of endorphins varies among individuals and can be influenced by factors such as genetics, fitness level, and the type of exercise undertaken. Moreover, while endorphins contribute significantly to the pleasurable sensations associated with physical activity, they are not the sole determinants of exercise's benefits. The broader spectrum of positive outcomes – from improved cardiovascular health to strengthened immunity – should be considered alongside the role of endorphins. As we delve further into the intricate workings of endorphins and their impact on our physiological and psychological well-being, it becomes increasingly evident that physical activity is a powerful catalyst for nurturing a healthier, more vibrant life. Embracing this knowledge allows us to appreciate the profound internal mechanisms at play when we lace up our sneakers or embark on an invigorating workout, reinforcing our commitment to leading an active and fulfilling lifestyle.

Personalizing Your Fitness Journey

Embarking on a fitness journey is a deeply personal and transformative experience. No two individuals are the same, and thus, no two fitness journeys will look exactly alike. Personalization in fitness is not just about tailoring the activities to suit your preferences, but also about aligning them with your unique strengths, weaknesses, and goals. This approach allows you to find joy and fulfillment in your fitness regimen, making it more sustainable and meaningful. When it comes to personalizing your fitness journey, self-reflection is key. Take the time to assess your current lifestyle, physical abilities, and mental well-being. Consider what motivates you, what brings you joy, and what challenges you. Understanding these aspects will help you craft a fitness plan that resonates with you on a deeper level. Another vital aspect of personalization involves setting realistic and attainable goals. These should be specific, measurable, and relevant to your aspirations. Whether it's improving endurance, building strength, or enhancing flexibility, defining clear objectives provides a roadmap for your fitness journey. Moreover, celebrating small victories along the way can serve as powerful motivation, fostering a sense of accomplishment and progress. Additionally, experimenting with various forms of exercise can uncover activities that truly resonate with you. From yoga and dance to hiking and weight training, exploring different options allows you to discover what ignites your passion and sustains your interest. Remember, the most effective fitness routine is one that you genuinely enjoy and eagerly anticipate. Personalizing your fitness journey also involves recognizing the importance of recovery and rest. Listening to your body and providing it with ample time for rejuvenation is essential for long-term well-being. Overexertion can lead to burnout and injury, hindering your progress and dampening your enthusiasm. Embracing balance is integral to sustainability. Finally, seeking support and guidance from a mentor, coach, or like-minded community can provide invaluable encouragement and accountability. Sharing experiences, receiving constructive feedback, and celebrating achievements with others can enrich your journey and reinforce your commitment to fitness. Remember, your fitness journey is a testament to your growth, resilience, and self-care. Embrace the process, celebrate every milestone, and cherish the personal transformation it brings.

Maintaining Motivation: A Heartfelt Guide

Maintaining motivation on your fitness journey is a deeply personal and emotional experience. It's natural to encounter hurdles and moments of doubt, but through sincere self-reflection and perseverance, you can keep the flame of motivation burning bright. Sometimes, it's not just about setting specific goals or reaching specific milestones. It's about finding meaning in the daily rituals of exercise and physical activity. The true essence of maintaining motivation lies in understanding that every step, no matter how small, contributes to your overall well-being. Each gentle yoga session, nature walk, or strength training session adds up to create a healthier, more vibrant you. Every moment of movement is an act of self-love. To maintain motivation, it's important to embrace the highs and lows of the journey. Celebrate your achievements no matter how small, and be gentle with yourself during challenging times. Surround yourself with a supportive community - whether it's a group exercise class, an online fitness forum, or friends who share your passion for well-being. Having a support system can provide encouragement and accountability when motivation wanes. Exploring new activities and settings can also reignite your passion for fitness. Whether it's hiking through serene forests, taking a refreshing swim in a crystal-clear lake, or joining a lively dance class, connecting with nature and trying new experiences can infuse vitality and enthusiasm into your routine. Remember, motivation is not a constant state, but an evolving journey. Embracing this truth allows you to appreciate the fluctuations in motivation as part of your growth. Lastly, always remind yourself of the intrinsic value of your efforts. Your dedication to taking care of your body and mind is a testament to your commitment to living a fulfilling life. In those moments when motivation seems elusive, tap into your inner strength and resilience. You are capable of achieving great things, and each small step forward is a triumph worthy of celebration.

Exploring Outdoor Activities for Well-being

Spending time outdoors not only rejuvenates the body, but it also nourishes the soul. Engaging in outdoor activities can have a profound impact on our overall well-being, providing a sense of tranquility and connectedness with nature. Whether it's going for a peaceful hike in the woods, enjoying a calming yoga session by the beach, or simply taking a leisurely stroll through a serene park, the outdoors offers endless opportunities for promoting physical and mental health. The fresh air, sunlight, and natural scenery create an environment that is conducive to relaxation and mindfulness, allowing us to escape from the hustle and bustle of daily life. Furthermore, outdoor activities often involve some degree of physical exercise, making them doubly beneficial for our health. By immersing ourselves in nature, we can find solace and inspiration, giving ourselves the opportunity to appreciate the beauty that surrounds us. This connection with nature acts as a powerful antidote to stress, anxiety, and fatigue, nurturing a sense of calm and inner peace. Additionally, participating in outdoor activities creates opportunities for social engagement, whether it's joining a community sports team, taking part in outdoor group fitness classes, or simply bonding with friends and family during a picnic in the park. These interactions foster a sense of belonging and support, contributing to our overall emotional well-being. Finally, embracing the great outdoors encourages us to adopt a more sustainable and eco-friendly lifestyle, instilling a deeper appreciation for the environment and the need to protect it. By embracing outdoor activities, we not only benefit our own well-being but also contribute to the preservation of our natural surroundings. Thus, let us venture out and immerse ourselves in the gifts that the outdoors has to offer, embracing the profound impact it can have on our holistic health and well-being.

Addressing Common Myths and Misconceptions

In the realm of exercise and physical activity, myths and misconceptions abound, often clouding the path to a healthier lifestyle. One common misconception is the belief that exercise is only effective if it leads to immediate weight loss. In reality, physical activity offers numerous benefits beyond shedding pounds, including improved cardiovascular health, enhanced mood, and increased energy levels.

Another prevalent myth is that one must engage in intense workouts to reap the rewards of exercise. The truth is that consistency and finding activities that bring joy and fulfillment are more impactful than pushing oneself to the limit. Additionally, there is a widespread misconception that exercise is only for the young and fit. On the contrary, individuals of all ages and fitness levels can benefit from regular physical activity, tailored to their capabilities and preferences. Yet another misconception is that certain body types are predisposed to excel in specific types of exercise. The reality is that with dedication and proper training, individuals of various body shapes and sizes can achieve remarkable progress in any form of physical activity. Moreover, there exists a mistaken belief that exercise is solely about sculpting the body and has little impact on mental well-being. Research demonstrates that physical activity not only enhances physical health but also contributes significantly to improved cognition, stress reduction, and overall emotional well-being. Lastly, the popular misconception persists that a busy schedule leaves no room for exercise. In truth, integrating small bursts of physical activity throughout the day, such as taking short walks or performing quick home workouts, can effectively support one's health goals. By dispelling these myths and misconceptions, individuals can approach exercise with a clearer mindset, paving the way for a more sustainable and fulfilling journey toward well-being.

Stories of Transformation: Inspiring Real-life Experiences

In this section, we delve into the awe-inspiring narratives of individuals whose lives have been profoundly impacted by embracing a fitness-focused lifestyle. These real-life accounts are not merely anecdotal evidence but serve as testaments to the incredible power of exercise and physical activity in transforming one's well-being. Through these gripping stories, we witness how individuals have overcome formidable challenges, restored their health, and found renewed purpose through the simple yet transformative act of engaging in regular physical activity. Each story is a poignant reminder that the journey towards physical wellness is often intertwined with profound emotional and mental breakthroughs. We encounter tales of individuals who, despite grappling with various health issues or sedentary lifestyles, courageously embarked on their exercise journeys, defying the limitations imposed upon them by others and themselves. These stories illustrate the remarkable resilience and determination that propel individuals to push beyond their perceived boundaries and achieve personal triumphs. At the heart of these narratives lies the revelation that exercise is not just a physical pursuit; it is a deeply emotional and psychological odyssey that empowers individuals to discover their inner strength and resilience. Moreover, these stories illuminate the diverse forms that transformation can take, transcending mere physical changes. Beyond weight loss and muscle gain, the transformations encompass a profound renewal of self-confidence, an alleviation of stress and anxiety, and a newfound zest for life. We witness the ripple effect of these individual transformations, as lives are buoyed by newfound energy and passion, radiating outwards to positively impact families, friends, and communities. Through these compelling accounts, readers are invited to empathize, learn, and draw inspiration from the lived experiences of these remarkable individuals. Their narratives bridge the gap between theory and reality, infusing the subject of exercise and physical activity with palpable human emotion, relatability, and hope. These are not embellished success stories, but authentic chronicles of everyday heroes who have embraced an active way of life and reaped extraordinary rewards in the process. It is our genuine hope that these stories resonate deeply with readers, instilling within them the unwavering belief that transformation is indeed within reach for anyone willing to embark on the transformative journey of exercise and physical activity.

Nutrition and Diet

The Connection Between Diet and Brain Health

A growing body of research suggests that our dietary choices play a crucial role in shaping brain health and cognitive function. The foods we consume not only fuel our bodies but also have a profound impact on the way our brains function. This connection between diet and brain health goes beyond just physical nourishment; it encompasses mental clarity, emotional well-being, and overall cognitive performance. When we delve into the intricate relationship between nutrition and brain health, we discover that certain dietary patterns can significantly influence mental clarity and cognitive function. For instance, a diet rich in whole foods, such as fruits, vegetables, whole grains, and lean proteins, provides essential nutrients like vitamins, minerals, and antioxidants that support optimal brain function. On the contrary, diets high in processed foods, sugars, and unhealthy fats have been linked to cognitive decline and an increased risk of neurodegenerative diseases. Additionally, exploring the benefits of specific nutrients such as omega-3 fatty acids, found in fatty fish and nuts, reveals their role in supporting cognitive function and maintaining brain health. As we uncover the impact of different dietary patterns, we gain valuable insights into how the foods we eat can either enhance or impair our cognitive abilities. This understanding empowers us to make informed choices about our diet, ultimately contributing to improved mental clarity and overall brain health.

Essential Nutrients for Cognitive Function

An optimal diet plays a crucial role in supporting cognitive function and overall brain health. Essential nutrients such as omega-3 fatty acids, antioxidants, vitamins, and minerals are fundamental in maintaining the intricate processes of the brain. Omega-3 fatty acids, found primarily in fish, flaxseeds, and walnuts, are renowned for their neuroprotective properties. These healthy fats have been associated with improved cognitive function, memory, and mood regulation. Additionally, antioxidants like vitamin E, vitamin C, and beta-carotene play a vital role in protecting brain cells from oxidative stress and inflammation. These nutrients can be sourced from a diverse range of fruits, vegetables, nuts, and seeds to support optimal brain function. Furthermore, B vitamins, particularly B6, B12, and folate, are essential for neurotransmitter synthesis and methylation processes within the brain, contributing to cognitive performance and emotional well-being. Minerals such as iron, zinc, and magnesium are also indispensable for neurotransmission, enzyme activity, and overall brain function. The incorporation of a balanced and varied diet rich in these essential nutrients is paramount for promoting cognitive resilience and reducing the risk of age-related cognitive decline. As we delve deeper into the significance of nutrition for the brain, it becomes evident that a mindful approach to dietary choices can profoundly impact cognitive function and mental clarity.

The Impact of Sugar and Processed Foods

Sugar and processed foods have become pervasive in modern diets, profoundly influencing not only our physical health but also our cognitive well-being. The detrimental effects of excessive sugar consumption on the brain are staggering. Research has shown that high sugar intake can lead to inflammation in the brain, impair cognitive function, and contribute to an increased risk of neurological disorders. Additionally, the rapid spikes and subsequent crashes in blood sugar levels caused by processed foods can disrupt the brain's energy supply, resulting in fatigue, mood swings, and difficulty concentrating. Moreover, the addictive nature of sugar can create a cycle of cravings and reward-seeking behavior, further exacerbating its impact on mental clarity and emotional stability. Processed foods, laden with artificial additives, preservatives, and trans fats, not only lack essential nutrients for cognitive support but also introduce harmful substances that can compromise brain health over time. The excessive consumption of these foods has been linked to a higher risk of cognitive decline, memory problems, and an increased susceptibility to developing neurodegenerative diseases. Understanding the profound impact of sugar and processed foods on the brain empowers individuals to make informed dietary choices that will positively influence their cognitive function and overall well-being. By recognizing the detrimental effects of these choices, one can take steps to reduce the intake of sugar and processed foods, thereby safeguarding and promoting long-term brain health. Embracing a diet rich in whole, unprocessed foods and mindful of added sugars can lead to improved cognitive performance, enhanced mood regulation, and a reduced risk of age-related cognitive decline.

Incorporating Antioxidant-Rich Foods

Antioxidants are compounds that can help neutralize free radicals in the body and protect cells from damage. When it comes to brain health, incorporating antioxidant-rich foods into your diet is essential for supporting cognitive function and overall well-being. These powerful nutrients can help reduce oxidative stress and inflammation, which are linked to various neurological conditions. To maximize your antioxidant intake, consider including a variety of colorful fruits and vegetables in your meals. Berries such as blueberries, strawberries, and raspberries are particularly rich in antioxidants like flavonoids and polyphenols. Additionally, vibrant vegetables like spinach, kale, and bell peppers contain high levels of vitamins C and E, two key antioxidants known for their protective effects on the brain. Other sources of antioxidants include nuts, seeds, and whole grains, which provide important minerals like selenium and copper that support the body's defense against oxidative damage. In addition to plant-based foods, certain herbs and spices like turmeric, cinnamon, and ginger boast potent antioxidant properties and can be easily incorporated into cooking. By making mindful choices about the foods you consume, you can proactively enhance your brain health and contribute to long-term cognitive vitality. Embracing an antioxidant-rich diet not only nourishes your body but also empowers you to take proactive steps in promoting mental clarity and emotional well-being.

The Role of Healthy Fats

Healthy fats play a crucial role in supporting brain health and cognitive function. Omega-3 fatty acids, found in abundance in certain foods such as salmon, mackerel, and flaxseeds, have been linked to improved mental clarity, focus, and memory. These essential fats are vital for the structure and function of brain cell membranes, promoting efficient communication between neurons and supporting neuroplasticity. Additionally, omega-3s have anti-inflammatory properties that can help protect the brain from damage and degeneration. Incorporating sources of monounsaturated and polyunsaturated fats, such as avocados, nuts, and olive oil, into your diet can also contribute to optimal brain health. These fats provide a sustainable source of energy for the brain and work to regulate cholesterol levels, reducing the risk of cardiovascular issues that can impact blood flow to the brain. In turn, this supports overall cognitive function and may lower the risk of cognitive decline. It's important to note that while healthy fats are beneficial for the brain, moderation is key. Aim to include these fats as part of a balanced diet, alongside a variety of fruits, vegetables, and lean proteins. By embracing a diverse range of nutrient-dense foods, you can optimize the overall nutritional support for your brain and body. Furthermore, research has shown that diets rich in healthy fats can positively influence mood and emotional well-being. By maintaining stable blood sugar levels and promoting the production of serotonin, the 'feel-good' neurotransmitter, these fats may contribute to a more balanced emotional state. This highlights the interconnected nature of nutrition and mental health, emphasizing the significance of nourishing both the body and mind. In conclusion, recognizing the importance of healthy fats in promoting brain health is an essential step towards establishing a holistic approach to well-being. By incorporating a variety of sources of healthy fats into your diet, you can support cognitive function, protect against age-related decline, and cultivate a sense of vitality that extends beyond physical health. Embracing the benefits of these essential nutrients is a valuable investment in your long-term brain health and overall quality of life.

Hydration and Brain Efficiency

Proper hydration is essential for maintaining optimal brain function and overall well-being. The human brain is composed of about 75% water, and even mild dehydration can significantly affect cognitive performance. When the body is dehydrated, it not only impacts the physical aspects such as endurance and coordination but also leads to a decline in mental focus, alertness, and memory retention. This emphasizes the critical importance of staying adequately hydrated throughout the day. Hydration plays a key role in regulating the brain's temperature, ensuring proper nutrient delivery, and removing waste products. Water is also involved in the production of neurotransmitters, the chemical messengers that facilitate communication between brain cells. Maintaining a state of optimal hydration supports the brain's ability to concentrate, process information, and maintain emotional stability. In addition to water, certain beverages and foods contribute to hydration. While water is the most efficient way to stay hydrated, consuming fruits, vegetables, and herbal teas can also contribute to fluid intake. However, it is important to be mindful of the consumption of sugary or caffeinated drinks, as excessive amounts of these can lead to dehydration due to their diuretic effects. Establishing a habit of regular, moderate water intake can be beneficial for brain efficiency. It is recommended to drink at least 8-10 glasses of water per day, but individual needs may vary based on factors such as climate, physical activity, and overall health. Monitoring urine color can serve as a practical indicator of hydration status - a pale yellow color generally indicates adequate hydration, while darker urine may signify the need for increased fluid intake. Furthermore, it's important to be mindful of staying hydrated not just during physical activities, but also throughout daily routines, work, and leisure time. Keeping a water bottle within reach and setting reminders to drink water can be helpful strategies for maintaining hydration levels. Small, consistent sips of water are often more effective than trying to consume large quantities all at once. By prioritizing proper hydration, individuals can enhance their cognitive abilities, sustain mental clarity, and promote overall brain efficiency. Making conscious choices to support hydration not only benefits immediate cognitive function but also contributes to long-term brain health and well-being.

Balancing Meals for Optimal Brain Performance

Achieving optimal brain performance is not just about what you eat, but also how you structure your meals. Balancing your meals to support cognitive function involves incorporating a variety of nutrients and food groups into your daily diet. Start by ensuring that each meal contains a combination of complex carbohydrates, lean proteins, healthy fats, and a rich array of vitamins and minerals. These components work synergistically to provide sustained energy and nourishment for your brain. Whole grains, such as brown rice and quinoa, are excellent sources of complex carbohydrates, which release glucose slowly into the bloodstream, providing a steady supply of energy to the brain. Pairing these carbohydrates with lean proteins, like chicken, fish, or tofu, can further stabilize blood sugar levels and enhance neurotransmitter function. Additionally, including healthy fats from sources like avocados, nuts, and olive oil can aid in optimizing brain health. These fats play a vital role in building cell membranes and supporting overall cognitive function. Remember to include a variety of colorful fruits and vegetables in your meals to benefit from their diverse range of antioxidants, vitamins, and minerals. Consuming a rainbow of produce ensures that you are supplying your brain with essential nutrients to combat oxidative stress and inflammation. Finally, don't forget the importance of hydration. Water is crucial for maintaining proper brain function, so be sure to drink an adequate amount throughout the day. By consciously designing well-rounded meals that encompass this spectrum of nutrients, you can effectively fuel your brain for peak performance and long-term health.

Understanding Dietary Supplements

Dietary supplements have become increasingly popular as people seek additional support for their overall health and well-being. When it comes to brain health, it's important to understand the role that supplements can play in supporting cognitive function and mental acuity. Before incorporating any dietary supplement into your routine, it's critical to consult with a healthcare professional to ensure that it aligns with your individual needs and doesn't interact with any existing medications or conditions. When selecting supplements for brain health, look for those that are backed by scientific research and third-party testing to verify potency and purity. Common supplements that are often associated with cognitive support include Omega-3 fatty acids, which are known for their anti-inflammatory properties that benefit brain function. Additionally, various B vitamins, such as B6, B9 (folate), and B12, are essential for neurotransmitter synthesis and nerve health. Antioxidants like vitamin C and E are believed to protect the brain from oxidative stress, while mineral supplements like magnesium may also contribute to neurological function.Regardless of the supplements chosen, it's crucial to remember that they should complement, rather than replace, a balanced diet. A nutrient-rich, whole-food-based diet should always be the foundation of any approach to brain health. While dietary supplements can offer valuable support, they should not serve as a substitute for healthy eating and lifestyle habits. Lastly, keep in mind that individual responses to supplements may vary, and it's important to monitor how your body and mind respond to any new additions to your routine. Our collective understanding of the effects of dietary supplements on brain health continues to evolve, so staying informed about the latest research and recommendations is vital to making informed choices.

Cultural and Lifestyle Considerations

Cultural and lifestyle factors play a significant role in shaping our dietary habits and ultimately influencing brain health. The diverse cultures around the world offer a rich tapestry of culinary traditions, each with its unique approach to nutrition. From the Mediterranean diet's focus on fresh produce and olive oil to the traditional Japanese emphasis on seafood and fermented foods, every cultural eating pattern offers valuable insights into promoting overall well-being, including cognitive function. Understanding and respecting different cultural perspectives on food can provide a holistic view of nourishment, which can be beneficial for brain health. When we consider lifestyle, it is important to recognize the impact of daily routines, social behaviors, and stress levels on dietary choices. For instance, the hectic pace of modern life in urban settings may lead to reliance on convenience or fast food, which may not always align with optimal brain nutrition. Furthermore, social gatherings and celebrations often center around specific foods that hold cultural or emotional significance, emphasizing the deeply ingrained connection between food and communal experiences. Acknowledging these influences can help individuals make mindful choices that support brain health while honoring cultural and social traditions. Moreover, ancestral eating patterns and heritage-based cuisines carry the wisdom of generations, reflecting a harmonious relationship with nature and an innate understanding of seasonal, locally-sourced ingredients. By embracing these time-honored practices, individuals can tap into the wealth of knowledge embedded within their cultural heritage to cultivate a brain-conscious approach to eating. Additionally, recognizing the impact of geographical and environmental factors, such as access to fresh produce or exposure to sunlight, underscores the intricate interplay between lifestyle, culture, and nutrition in nurturing brain wellness. Ultimately, integrating cultural and lifestyle considerations into dietary choices empowers individuals to create a sustainable and fulfilling relationship with food that honors both personal and collective histories. Embracing diversity and traditional wisdom paves the way for a nourishing, brain-healthy diet that extends beyond physical nourishment, encompassing emotional, social, and cultural well-being.

Creating a Sustainable Eating Plan

As we continue to delve into the importance of nutrition for brain health, it becomes evident that a sustainable eating plan is not only beneficial for our physical well-being but also plays a crucial role in supporting cognitive function. Creating a sustainable eating plan involves thoughtful consideration of various factors, including personal preferences, cultural influences, and environmental impact. One key aspect of a sustainable eating plan is to prioritize whole, unprocessed foods that are nutrient-dense and environmentally friendly. This means choosing a variety of fruits, vegetables, whole grains, and legumes that are sustainably sourced whenever possible. By focusing on plant-based foods, individuals can reduce their carbon footprint while obtaining essential nutrients for brain health. In addition to food choices, portion control and mindful eating practices contribute to the sustainability of an individual's dietary habits. By being attentive to hunger cues and practicing moderation, individuals can reduce food waste and support their body's nutritional needs without overconsumption. Moreover, incorporating local and seasonal produce fosters a connection with the community and reduces the resources required for transportation and preservation. Furthermore, considering the long-term impact of dietary choices on personal well-being and the environment is vital when creating a sustainable eating plan. This entails taking into account the ethical and ecological implications of food production and consumption. For instance, opting for organic or ethically sourced products can promote sustainable agricultural practices and contribute to a healthier ecosystem. Integrating a sustainable eating plan into one's lifestyle also involves meal planning and preparation. Through careful meal planning, individuals can minimize food waste, save time and money, and ensure that they have access to nourishing meals throughout the week. By preparing homemade meals using fresh, wholesome ingredients, individuals can exercise control over the nutritional content of their food while aligning with sustainable practices. Embracing the concept of a sustainable eating plan goes beyond individual health; it extends to the well-being of the planet and future generations. By making conscious choices and adopting sustainable dietary habits, individuals can contribute to a more resilient and environmentally conscious food system. As we explore the intricate relationship between nutrition and sustainability, it becomes evident that thoughtful and informed dietary decisions have the power to positively impact both personal health and the world at large.

Medical Insights and Treatments

Understanding Medical Interventions

Medical interventions encompass a broad spectrum of treatments and procedures designed to address various health conditions and improve overall well-being. These interventions may range from simple preventative measures to complex surgical procedures, each tailored to meet the specific needs of the individual. The primary goal of medical interventions is to alleviate symptoms, manage chronic conditions, and in many cases, cure diseases. By gaining an understanding of these interventions, individuals can make informed decisions about their healthcare. It is essential to recognize that medical interventions are not only limited to traditional Western medicine but also encompass integrative and holistic approaches that focus on the mind-body connection. Understanding the purpose behind medical interventions is crucial in appreciating the potential outcomes they aim to achieve. For instance, some interventions may target the root cause of a condition, while others may focus on symptom management or disease prevention. Additionally, the effectiveness of medical interventions can vary based on factors such as the individual's overall health, genetic predispositions, and lifestyle choices. Moreover, medical interventions serve to empower individuals to take an active role in their health by providing access to diverse treatment options and resources. As the field of healthcare continues to evolve, medical interventions constantly adapt and improve, offering new hope and possibilities for those seeking medical support. It is important to approach the topic of medical interventions with an open mind, embracing the diversity of available treatments and considering the potential benefits for one's health and well-being.

Diagnostic Tools and Techniques

In the realm of understanding the intricacies of the brain, the utilization of advanced diagnostic tools and techniques plays a paramount role in enabling healthcare professionals to accurately assess neurological conditions. Magnetic Resonance Imaging (MRI) stands as one of the most crucial diagnostic tools for examining the structure and functionality of the brain. By providing detailed images, it allows for the identification of abnormalities such as tumors, lesions, or vascular malformations. Complementing MRI, Positron Emission Tomography (PET) scans help in visualizing metabolic activity, aiding in the detection of conditions like Alzheimer's disease and epilepsy. Another invaluable diagnostic technique, Electroencephalography (EEG), records the brain's electrical activity, facilitating the diagnosis of seizures, sleep disorders, and brain injuries. Furthermore, advancements in neuroimaging technologies have given rise to functional MRI (fMRI) and diffusion tensor imaging (DTI), which provide insights into brain function, connectivity, and white matter integrity. Such breakthroughs have revolutionized the ability to map neural networks and analyze brain circuitry, offering profound implications for understanding cognitive processes and identifying abnormalities associated with various neurological disorders. Additionally, advancements in genetic testing and biomarker analysis have opened new frontiers in diagnostic precision, allowing for personalized medicine and early intervention in conditions with genetic predispositions. It is crucial to highlight the significance of these diagnostic tools and techniques in potentially uncovering manifestations of neurological disorders at their earliest stages, thereby enhancing the prospects for effective treatment and management. The convergence of cutting-edge imaging technologies, genetic profiling, and innovative biomarker assays propels the advancements in diagnosing and understanding neurological conditions, instilling hope for improved prognoses and quality of life for individuals impacted by such disorders. With continuous strides in diagnostic innovation, the path towards early identification and targeted intervention becomes increasingly promising, signifying a monumental leap forward in the field of neurology.

Medications and Their Role

When it comes to managing various neurological conditions, medications play a crucial role in alleviating symptoms and improving the quality of life for individuals. Understanding the importance and nuances of different medications is essential for both patients and caregivers. Medications prescribed for neurological disorders are designed to address specific symptoms, such as tremors, cognitive decline, or mood disturbances. It's important to note that these medications can vary widely based on the condition being treated. Some drugs may target neurotransmitters in the brain to facilitate communication between cells, while others focus on reducing inflammation or modulating neural activity. The effectiveness of medications can also differ from person to person, and finding the right balance often requires close collaboration between patients, physicians, and specialists. Patients should be well-informed about the potential side effects and benefits of each medication, as well as any lifestyle adjustments that may be necessary. Additionally, understanding the importance of adherence to medication schedules and closely following dosage instructions cannot be overstated. Communicating openly and honestly with healthcare providers about any concerns, experiences with the medication, or observed changes is vital for optimizing treatment outcomes. Furthermore, exploring complementary therapies and lifestyle modifications alongside medications can offer a comprehensive approach to symptom management. Open conversations with healthcare professionals about alternative treatments and their potential interactions with prescribed medications can lead to more personalized care plans. Overall, medications are an integral part of the multifaceted approach to treating neurological conditions, and their role should be appreciated within the context of holistic care and individualized needs.

Therapeutic Approaches Explained

In this section, we delve into the various therapeutic approaches that are employed in the realm of brain health and wellness. Therapeutic interventions aim to enhance cognitive function, alleviate symptoms of neurological disorders, and improve overall mental well-being. One of the most widely recognized therapeutic approaches is cognitive-behavioral therapy (CBT), which focuses on identifying and modifying negative thought patterns and behaviors that may contribute to emotional distress or cognitive dysfunction. This approach has shown promising results in managing conditions such as anxiety, depression, and certain neurological disorders. Another crucial therapeutic approach is neurofeedback, a non-invasive technique that allows individuals to self-regulate their brain function by receiving real-time feedback on their brainwave activity. Neurofeedback has been increasingly utilized to address issues related to attention, stress management, and cognitive performance. Additionally, mindfulness-based therapies have gained prominence for their efficacy in promoting mental clarity, emotional resilience, and overall brain health. These approaches encompass mindfulness meditation, yoga, and other contemplative practices that train individuals to cultivate present-moment awareness and compassion. Furthermore, expressive therapies, including art therapy, music therapy, and dance/movement therapy, have been instrumental in providing avenues for self-expression, emotional processing, and psychological healing. These modalities offer individuals creative and sensorimotor outlets to communicate and explore their thoughts, emotions, and experiences, contributing to improved neural connectivity and emotional regulation. Moreover, emerging advancements in technology have paved the way for innovative therapeutic tools such as virtual reality (VR) therapy, which immerses individuals in simulated environments to address phobias, PTSD, and other cognitive challenges. Equally significant are the holistic approaches that integrate physical, emotional, and spiritual aspects of well-being, emphasizing the interconnectedness of mind and body. These modalities encompass acupuncture, herbal medicine, aromatherapy, and other alternative practices that aim to restore balance and harmony within the individual. The field of therapeutic approaches continues to evolve with ongoing research and multidisciplinary collaboration, paving the way for personalized, comprehensive care that addresses the diverse needs and preferences of individuals seeking to optimize their brain health and cognitive potential.

Integrative and Holistic Treatments

Integrative and holistic treatments encompass a diverse array of approaches aimed at addressing an individual's health from a comprehensive standpoint. These treatments often incorporate both traditional medical interventions and alternative therapies to promote overall well-being. At their core, integrative and holistic treatments focus on the interconnectedness of the body, mind, and spirit, acknowledging that optimal health arises from a harmonious balance among these elements. One key feature of these treatments is their emphasis on personalized care. Practitioners in this field recognize that each person's health profile is unique, and as such, treatment plans are tailored to address the specific needs and circumstances of the individual. This individualized approach may involve a combination of conventional medicine, such as prescription medications or surgical procedures, alongside complementary practices like acupuncture, chiropractic care, or herbal remedies. Furthermore, holistic treatments place a strong emphasis on preventive strategies and lifestyle modifications. This may include dietary changes, stress-reducing techniques, mindfulness practices, and physical exercises tailored to the individual's abilities and preferences. By nurturing healthy habits and proactively addressing potential health challenges, individuals can work towards achieving lasting wellness. Another fundamental aspect of integrative and holistic treatments is their focus on treating the root causes of ailments rather than merely alleviating symptoms. Through exploring the interconnected factors that contribute to an individual's health, practitioners seek to uncover underlying imbalances or dysfunctions. By addressing these root causes, individuals may experience more profound and sustainable improvements in their well-being. It is important to note that the effectiveness of integrative and holistic treatments often stems from a collaborative approach. Healthcare professionals in this field frequently work in interdisciplinary teams, sharing insights and drawing upon diverse perspectives to optimize patient care. This collaborative model fosters a supportive environment where individuals can benefit from the combined expertise of multiple practitioners, promoting holistic healing. As we delve into the realm of integrative and holistic treatments, it becomes apparent that these approaches not only aim to treat specific ailments but also strive to nurture an individual's overall vitality. By integrating various modalities and viewing health through a holistic lens, these treatments endeavor to empower individuals to embark on a journey towards enhanced well-being, resilience, and harmony.

Managing Chronic Conditions

Managing chronic conditions involves a comprehensive and multi-faceted approach that addresses the physical, emotional, and psychological aspects of the illness. It requires a partnership between healthcare providers and patients to develop personalized strategies aimed at enhancing quality of life and minimizing the impact of the condition on daily activities. Embracing a proactive mindset is essential, empowering individuals with chronic conditions to take an active role in their own care and well-being. This often begins with education and understanding the nature of the condition, including its triggers, symptoms, and potential complications. With this knowledge, individuals can develop effective coping mechanisms and make informed decisions regarding their lifestyle, treatment options, and self-care routines. One crucial aspect of managing chronic conditions is creating a support network encompassing healthcare professionals, family members, and peers who can provide empathy, encouragement, and practical assistance. The emotional toll of living with a chronic illness should not be underestimated, and having a strong support system can significantly alleviate feelings of isolation and despair. Moreover, peer support groups offer invaluable opportunities for individuals to share experiences, strategies, and resources, fostering a sense of community and empowerment. In addition to emotional support, managing chronic conditions also entails adhering to prescribed medical regimens, such as medication protocols and treatment plans. Adherence to these regimens is vital, as it directly impacts the efficacy of interventions and the progression of the condition. Integrating complementary therapies, such as acupuncture, yoga, or meditation, may also contribute to symptom management and overall well-being. However, it is imperative to consult healthcare professionals before incorporating these practices into one's routine to ensure compatibility with existing treatments. Furthermore, maintaining a healthy lifestyle through regular physical activity, balanced nutrition, and adequate sleep is paramount in effectively managing chronic conditions. Engaging in appropriate exercise routines not only promotes physical wellness but also enhances mental clarity and emotional resilience. Similarly, consuming a nutrient-dense diet rich in fruits, vegetables, lean proteins, and whole grains can bolster the body's immune system and foster optimal functioning. Adequate rest and relaxation are equally crucial, as they facilitate recuperation and help mitigate the stress that often accompanies chronic illnesses. Ultimately, managing chronic conditions is an ongoing journey that necessitates resilience, adaptability, and perseverance. By integrating various approaches that address the physical, emotional, and lifestyle dimensions of the condition, individuals can cultivate a holistic framework for navigating the challenges posed by chronic illness. This multifaceted approach empowers individuals to lead meaningful and fulfilling lives despite the constraints imposed by their conditions.

The Impact of Nutrition on Treatment Efficacy

Nutrition plays a crucial role in the efficacy and success of medical treatments, especially when it comes to managing chronic conditions. The foods we consume can have a direct impact on our body's ability to respond to various interventions, from medications to therapeutic approaches. Understanding the intricate relationship between nutrition and treatment efficacy is essential for individuals seeking to optimize their overall well-being and health outcomes. A balanced and nutrient-rich diet provides the body with the necessary building blocks for cellular repair, immune function, and overall vitality. When faced with chronic illnesses, the body's nutritional requirements may shift, making it imperative to pay close attention to dietary choices. For instance, individuals undergoing certain medical treatments may need to ensure adequate intake of specific nutrients that support the body's healing processes. Moreover, an optimal nutritional status can enhance the body's resilience and ability to tolerate certain medical interventions, potentially reducing the occurrence of adverse effects. In contrast, poor dietary habits can compromise the effectiveness of treatments, leading to suboptimal outcomes and prolonged recovery periods. Specific nutrients such as vitamins, minerals, antioxidants, and omega-3 fatty acids have been shown to exert profound effects on the body's response to medical therapies. For instance, vitamin D is known to play a crucial role in supporting immune function, which is particularly relevant for individuals undergoing treatments that may suppress the immune system. Similarly, the anti-inflammatory properties of certain foods can complement the management of conditions characterized by persistent inflammation. The synergy between nutrition and treatment efficacy extends beyond mere sustenance, encompassing the psychological and emotional aspects of healing. A wholesome diet can positively influence mental well-being, promoting a sense of empowerment and resilience in the face of medical challenges. Furthermore, the act of mindful eating and nourishing the body can instill a sense of control and optimism, fostering a conducive environment for successful treatment outcomes. By recognizing the profound impact of nutrition on treatment efficacy, individuals can proactively integrate dietary considerations into their overall healthcare strategy. Consultation with healthcare professionals, including registered dietitians and integrated medicine practitioners, can provide invaluable guidance in tailoring dietary plans to complement specific treatment regimens. Embracing this holistic approach to health empowers individuals to become active participants in their own healing journey, fostering an environment where treatments can achieve their maximal potential.

Patient Experiences and Perspectives

As we delve into the realm of medical insights and treatments, it is essential to explore the profound impact of patient experiences on the journey to wellness. Every individual navigating a health challenge has a unique story to tell, shaped by their encounters with healthcare providers, treatment regimens, and the resilience they display in the face of adversity. Patient experiences serve as invaluable sources of wisdom for both fellow patients and healthcare professionals. By sharing their stories, individuals shed light on the emotional and physical toll of their conditions, encapsulating the triumphs and tribulations that accompany their pursuit of healing. These narratives offer glimpses into the human side of medicine, allowing others to find solace in relatable accounts and offering insights that cannot be gleaned from clinical studies alone. Beyond the tangible aspects of treatment, patient perspectives provide a profound understanding of the holistic impact of illness. By articulating their challenges, hopes, and fears, individuals reveal the intricate interplay between the body, mind, and spirit. Their accounts underscore the importance of compassionate care, empathy, and effective communication in fostering healing environments where patients feel understood, valued, and empowered in their own care. Moreover, patient experiences elucidate the significance of personalized healthcare approaches. Each individual's journey reflects the diverse responses to various treatments, emphasizing the need for tailored interventions that honor the uniqueness of every patient. By embracing these narratives, healthcare professionals are better equipped to design comprehensive care plans that align with their patients' values, preferences, and aspirations. Despite the hardships they endure, many individuals convey remarkable resilience, offering inspiration and encouragement to others grappling with similar challenges. Their courage and determination exemplify the human capacity to navigate adversity and find purpose amidst trials. By sharing these narratives, they ignite hope and solidarity within the community while exemplifying the transformative power of the human spirit. In recognition of these profound contributions, this chapter seeks to honor and amplify the voices of those who have weathered the storm of illness, showcasing the beauty and strength inherent in their lived experiences.

Consulting Healthcare Professionals

Seeking guidance and support from healthcare professionals during your journey to better brain health is crucial. Whether you are managing a chronic condition, seeking treatment options, or simply aiming to optimize your overall well-being, consulting with the appropriate medical experts can provide invaluable insights and personalized recommendations. When approaching healthcare professionals, it's important to articulate your concerns, symptoms, and goals clearly and honestly. This transparency allows them to understand your specific needs and tailor their advice accordingly. Keep in mind that every individual's situation is unique, and effective communication serves as the foundation for fruitful interactions with healthcare providers. Depending on your requirements, various specialists may become instrumental in your care plan. Neurologists specialize in addressing conditions related to the nervous system, including the brain, spinal cord, and nerves, while psychiatrists focus on mental health aspects and psychological well-being. Additionally, nutritionists and dietitians can offer valuable insights into the impact of diet on brain function and overall cognitive health. In the realm of holistic healthcare, integrative medicine practitioners combine conventional medicine with alternative therapies to offer comprehensive and personalized treatment approaches. Their expertise encompasses a wide range of disciplines, including acupuncture, massage therapy, and mindfulness practices, among others. Collaborating with these professionals can contribute to a well-rounded and holistic approach to brain health. Furthermore, once you've established a relationship with your healthcare team, maintaining regular check-ins and follow-ups is essential for monitoring your progress and making any necessary adjustments to your treatment plan. Embracing a proactive role in your healthcare journey empowers you to actively participate in decision-making processes and ensures that your concerns are addressed effectively. Always remember that healthcare professionals are eager to collaborate with you in enhancing your brain health and overall well-being. By fostering open and honest communication, building trust, and embracing their expert guidance, you can navigate your path to improved brain health with confidence and optimism.

Navigating the Path to Recovery

Navigating the path to recovery can be a complex and challenging journey, often requiring patience, perseverance, and the guidance of healthcare professionals. It's essential to recognize that recovery is a unique and highly individualized process, influenced by a myriad of factors such as the nature of the condition, personal circumstances, and the availability of support systems. As individuals embark on this journey, it's important for them to maintain an open dialogue with their healthcare team, sharing their concerns, fears, and triumphs along the way. Recovery often involves setting achievable goals, both short-term and long-term, that align with the individual's capabilities and aspirations. These objectives may encompass physical rehabilitation, emotional well-being, lifestyle adjustments, or cultivating a positive mindset. Moreover, acknowledging setbacks as normal components of the recovery process can help individuals build resilience and determination. In addition to medical interventions, the provision of holistic care plays a crucial role in recovery. This encompasses not only physical health but also mental and emotional well-being. It involves fostering supportive relationships, engaging in meaningful activities, and adopting self-care practices. These aspects can contribute significantly to an individual's overall sense of wellness and aid in their journey toward recovery. Throughout the recovery process, it's fundamental for individuals to remain informed about their condition and treatment options. This empowers them to actively participate in decision-making regarding their health and well-being. Seeking out reliable sources of information, asking pertinent questions, and collaborating closely with healthcare professionals can facilitate a sense of control and autonomy throughout the recovery trajectory. Another pivotal aspect of navigating the path to recovery involves embracing a proactive mindset. This entails cultivating a positive outlook, drawing on inner strengths, and believing in the possibility of improvement and healing. Studies have shown the profound impact of a positive attitude on the recovery process, highlighting the significance of cultivating hope and optimism during challenging times. Furthermore, social support and community engagement are invaluable components of recovery. Connecting with understanding peers, support groups, or mentorship programs can provide solace, inspiration, and practical advice. Sharing experiences and insights with others who have walked similar paths can foster a sense of belonging and encourage individuals to persevere despite the obstacles they may encounter. As individuals navigate their path to recovery, it's essential for them to practice self-compassion and patience. Acknowledging personal progress, no matter how incremental, and celebrating small victories along the way can bolster resilience and motivation. Each step taken in the direction of recovery, no matter how small, is a testament to one's strength and determination. In conclusion, the path to recovery is marked by its ups and downs, yet it holds the promise of renewal and restored well-being. By embracing a collaborative approach with healthcare professionals, setting realistic goals, nurturing holistic wellness, staying informed, fostering resilience, maintaining positivity, seeking support, and practicing self-compassion, individuals can navigate their path to recovery with greater confidence and resilience.

Recent Scientific Studies

Introduction to Recent Research

In the realm of neuroscientific research, recent advancements have propelled our understanding of the brain to unprecedented heights. Breakthrough discoveries in neurology have fundamentally shifted our perception of brain function and capacity, ushering in an era of immense potential for improving human health and cognition. The significance of recent research cannot be overstated; it illuminates the intricate mechanisms that underpin our cognitive processes and emotional experiences. As we delve into the realms of neuroplasticity, memory formation, and neurological disorders, each new finding serves as a building block for further exploration and development. It is through these scientific revelations that we gain insight into the astonishing complexity and adaptability of the human brain. The implications of these findings reach far beyond the confines of the laboratory, touching the lives of individuals grappling with neurological conditions and paving the way for innovative treatment modalities. To comprehend the impact of recent research is to grasp the boundless potential for enhancing human well-being and unlocking the mysteries of the mind.

Breakthrough Discoveries in Neurology

In the ever-evolving landscape of neurology, there have been remarkable breakthroughs that have revolutionized our understanding of the human brain. Recent advancements in various neuroscientific disciplines have paved the way for unprecedented insights and transformative possibilities in addressing neurological conditions. One such breakthrough pertains to the field of neuroimaging, where state-of-the-art techniques such as functional magnetic resonance imaging (fMRI) and positron emission tomography (PET) scans have provided a window into the intricate workings of the brain. These cutting-edge technologies have allowed researchers to observe neural activity with unprecedented precision, unraveling the complexities of neurological disorders and offering potential diagnostic and treatment avenues. Additionally, the emergence of optogenetics, a novel interdisciplinary approach, has enabled scientists to manipulate neuronal activity with light, unveiling new pathways for understanding the neural circuitry underlying various cognitive processes. The fusion of computational neuroscience and machine learning has delivered groundbreaking computational models that simulate brain functions, fostering revolutionary insights into the mechanisms governing perception, decision-making, and memory. Moreover, the integration of genetics and epigenetics has unearthed crucial genetic determinants of neurological diseases, shedding light on personalized treatment strategies and approaching neurodegenerative disorders with heightened precision and specificity. Collectively, these breakthrough discoveries have reshaped the contours of neurology, propelling the field towards innovative interventions and holistic perspectives on brain health. The profound implications of these advances reverberate across diverse domains, from clinical practice to public health policy, opening doors to a future where neurological conditions can be understood, managed, and mitigated with unprecedented efficacy and compassion.

Understanding Memory and Learning

Memory and learning are fundamental aspects of human cognition, deeply intertwined with our ability to navigate the world around us. As we explore the intricate workings of the brain, we uncover the remarkable processes involved in memory formation and learning acquisition. Memories are not static entities but are continuously molded, updated, and reinterpreted by our experiences. Neuroplasticity, the brain's remarkable ability to reorganize itself by forming new neural connections throughout life, plays a crucial role in shaping our memories and influencing our capacity to learn. When we engage in learning activities, whether through education, practical experiences, or skill development, our neurons forge new pathways and strengthen existing connections. This process is essential for acquiring knowledge and skills and plays a significant role in cognitive development. Furthermore, the consolidation of long-term memories depends on complex interactions between various brain regions, including the hippocampus and the prefrontal cortex. Understanding this interplay provides valuable insights into how we encode, store, and retrieve information. However, the topic of memory and learning extends beyond the biological aspects. Psychological factors such as attention, motivation, and emotional significance profoundly influence memory formation and learning outcomes. Emotions, for instance, can enhance or distort our recollection of events, demonstrating the intricate relationship between cognition and affective experiences. In addition, individual differences in memory and learning abilities underscore the uniqueness of each person's cognitive profile. Some individuals may exhibit exceptional memory capabilities, while others excel in specific types of learning tasks. Recognizing and embracing these diversities can enrich educational practices and contribute to a more inclusive approach to learning. Advancements in neuroscience have also shed light on the potential implications for improving memory and learning, offering promising avenues for interventions and enhancements. Cognitive training, memory techniques, and educational strategies informed by neuroscientific research hold the potential to optimize learning outcomes and support cognitive well-being across diverse populations. As we delve deeper into the enigmatic realm of memory and learning, we unravel the interconnectedness of neural processes, psychological phenomena, and environmental influences. By embracing a multidimensional understanding of memory and learning, we can harness this knowledge to foster intellectual growth, adaptability, and the pursuit of lifelong learning.

The Science of Neuroplasticity

Neuroplasticity, also known as brain plasticity, has revolutionized our understanding of the human brain's incredible adaptability and capacity for change. This phenomenon reveals that the brain is not a fixed entity but rather a highly dynamic and malleable organ capable of reorganizing itself in response to new experiences, learning, or injuries. Understanding neuroplasticity offers profound insights into how we can enhance cognitive abilities, recover from brain injuries, and even mitigate the impact of neurological disorders. It is an awe-inspiring testament to the resilience and potential inherent in the human brain. Research in neuroplasticity has demonstrated that the brain retains its ability to create new neural connections and pathways throughout life, challenging the long-held belief that the brain's structure remains relatively static after a certain age. This means that individuals can actively nurture and stimulate their brain's plasticity through various activities, including cognitive exercises, learning new skills, engaging in creative pursuits, and maintaining a stimulating environment. Furthermore, neuroplasticity is foundational in neurorehabilitation, offering hope and promise to individuals recovering from strokes, traumatic brain injuries, or neurodegenerative diseases. By harnessing the brain's adaptive capabilities, therapists and healthcare professionals can develop innovative interventions to facilitate recovery and improve quality of life for patients. Moreover, ongoing research in neuroplasticity has revealed the potential for developing targeted therapies to address conditions such as chronic pain, post-traumatic stress disorder, and autism spectrum disorders. The implications of neuroplasticity extend beyond individual advancements to inform educational practices, organizational management strategies, and societal approaches to mental health and well-being. Embracing the principles of neuroplasticity can empower individuals to adopt a growth mindset, cultivate resilience, and strive for continuous personal development. As we delve deeper into the complexities of neuroplasticity, we uncover the remarkable capacities of the human brain to adapt, learn, and thrive amidst the ever-changing landscape of life's experiences.

Advancements in Brain Health Technologies

In recent years, the field of neuroscience has witnessed remarkable advancements in the realm of brain health technologies. These innovations have revolutionized our understanding of the brain and have opened up new frontiers in the diagnosis and treatment of neurological disorders. One such breakthrough is the development of non-invasive imaging techniques, such as functional magnetic resonance imaging (fMRI) and positron emission tomography (PET), which allow researchers to observe brain activity in real time. These tools have provided invaluable insights into the mechanisms underlying various cognitive functions, paving the way for more targeted interventions. Alongside imaging technologies, the rise of neurostimulation devices has offered promising prospects for addressing conditions like chronic pain, depression, and epilepsy. Techniques like transcranial magnetic stimulation (TMS) and deep brain stimulation (DBS) have shown significant potential in modulating neural circuits and alleviating symptoms in individuals with treatment-resistant neurological conditions. Furthermore, the integration of artificial intelligence (AI) and machine learning has enhanced the precision and efficiency of diagnostic procedures. AI algorithms can analyze complex neuroimaging data and identify patterns indicative of neurological diseases with a level of accuracy that was previously unattainable. This not only expedites the diagnostic process but also facilitates early intervention, leading to improved patient outcomes. Moreover, wearable technologies equipped with biosensors have empowered individuals to monitor their brain health in real time. These devices can track vital metrics, such as brain wave patterns and sleep quality, providing users with actionable insights to optimize their cognitive well-being. As the pace of innovation accelerates, the convergence of brain health technologies with personalized medicine holds immense promise for tailoring treatments to individual neurobiological profiles. This paradigm shift towards precision therapeutics has the potential to revolutionize how we approach brain-related illnesses, ushering in an era of customized, patient-centric care. The ongoing evolution of these technologies not only augments our understanding of the brain but also underscores the transformative impact they can have on enhancing the lives of those affected by neurological conditions.

Cognitive Decline: New Insights

Cognitive decline, often associated with aging, has long been a topic of concern and interest within the field of neuroscience. As our population continues to grow older, the prevalence of cognitive disorders, such as dementia and Alzheimer's disease, has become increasingly prominent. In this section, we will explore the latest insights and research findings related to cognitive decline, shedding light on the complexities of these conditions and the potential avenues for intervention. Understanding the underlying mechanisms of cognitive decline is crucial for developing effective preventive measures and treatments. Recent studies have revealed compelling evidence linking lifestyle factors, such as diet, exercise, and social engagement, to cognitive health. The role of neuroplasticity in mitigating cognitive decline has garnered significant attention, offering hope for novel therapeutic approaches. Moreover, advancements in brain imaging techniques have provided unprecedented insights into the structural and functional changes associated with cognitive impairment, allowing for early detection and targeted interventions. One area of particular interest is the impact of chronic stress on cognitive function. Research has shown that prolonged exposure to stress hormones can detrimentally affect brain regions involved in memory and decision-making, contributing to accelerated cognitive decline. Understanding the intricate interplay between stress and cognitive health can inform strategies for stress management and resilience-building, potentially mitigating the risk of cognitive impairment in vulnerable populations. Furthermore, emerging studies have underscored the importance of addressing cardiovascular health as a foundational aspect of preserving cognitive function. The close relationship between heart health and brain health highlights the significance of managing risk factors such as hypertension, diabetes, and obesity in maintaining cognitive vitality. These findings emphasize the holistic nature of cognitive decline and the need for integrated healthcare approaches that consider both physical and mental well-being. In examining new insights into cognitive decline, it is essential to recognize the profound impact on individuals, families, and society as a whole. The growing body of knowledge surrounding cognitive disorders instills a sense of urgency in pursuing multifaceted strategies to support cognitive resilience and enhance the quality of life for those affected. By delving into the forefront of scientific inquiry, we endeavor to illuminate pathways toward a future where cognitive decline is met with understanding, innovation, and compassion.

Research on Mental Health Disorders

Mental health disorders have always been a significant area of research and understanding when it comes to the brain. The intricacies of conditions such as depression, anxiety, bipolar disorder, schizophrenia, and many others continue to challenge scientists and researchers. Recent studies have shed light on the biological, environmental, and genetic factors that contribute to the onset and progression of these disorders. Understanding the underlying mechanisms of mental health conditions is crucial for developing effective treatments and interventions. Advancements in neuroscience have allowed for a deeper exploration of the neural correlates of mental illnesses. For instance, neuroimaging techniques such as functional Magnetic Resonance Imaging (fMRI) have enabled researchers to observe the differences in brain activity and connectivity among individuals with various mental health disorders compared to those without. Additionally, the role of neurotransmitters and neurochemical imbalances in contributing to these conditions has been a subject of extensive research. Studies focusing on the impact of early-life experiences, trauma, and stress on brain development and susceptibility to mental health disorders have also provided invaluable insights. Furthermore, the exploration of epigenetic influences on gene expression related to mental health has opened new avenues for understanding the interplay between genetics and environment. Research into the effectiveness of various therapies, including medication, psychotherapy, and holistic approaches, continues to be a vital part of addressing mental health disorders. Moreover, recent studies have emphasized the importance of personalized treatment plans tailored to an individual's specific neurobiological and psychological makeup. Through collaborative efforts between neuroscientists, psychiatrists, psychologists, and other healthcare professionals, there is a growing understanding that mental health disorders are complex and multifaceted conditions that require comprehensive and compassionate care. The ethical considerations surrounding research in this field, such as informed consent, privacy, and the potential implications of new interventions, continue to be critical areas of examination. As we navigate through the expanding landscape of mental health research, it becomes increasingly evident that a holistic approach acknowledging both the biological and environmental influences is essential for promoting mental well-being and resilience. The ongoing dedication of researchers and practitioners worldwide to advance our understanding of mental health disorders is paving the way for more effective strategies to support individuals in their recovery journeys.

The Role of AI in Neuroscience

The intersection of artificial intelligence and neuroscience presents a promising frontier in the exploration of the human brain. As technology continues to advance, AI has increasingly become a valuable tool in elucidating the complex workings of the brain. Through sophisticated algorithms and machine learning, AI offers new perspectives on understanding neural networks, synaptic connections, and cognitive processes. By analyzing large datasets and identifying patterns that may elude human perception, AI enables researchers to delve deeper into brain functioning than ever before. One of the most compelling applications of AI in neuroscience is in the field of neuroimaging. Advanced imaging techniques combined with AI algorithms allow for more precise and detailed analysis of brain structure and function. This not only aids in the diagnosis and treatment of neurological disorders but also provides deeper insights into the mechanisms underlying various cognitive functions. Furthermore, AI plays a pivotal role in modeling and simulating neural systems. Complex computational models powered by AI enable scientists to simulate the behavior of neural circuits, offering a virtual platform to test hypotheses and explore potential treatments for neurological conditions. These simulations allow researchers to observe how neural networks respond to stimuli and how different parameters can influence brain activity, providing invaluable information for developing targeted interventions. In addition, AI contributes to the development of innovative neuroprosthetic devices and brain-computer interfaces. By leveraging AI's capability for real-time data analysis and interpretation, these technologies hold the potential to restore mobility and communication for individuals with brain injuries or neurodegenerative diseases. The integration of AI with neuroscience opens doors to creating more effective interventions and improving the quality of life for those affected by neurological challenges. However, as with any powerful technology, the ethical considerations pertaining to the use of AI in neuroscience cannot be overlooked. Questions regarding privacy, security, and informed consent emerge as AI-driven tools expand in the realm of brain research. Maintaining ethical standards and safeguarding against misuse of AI-generated insights are crucial aspects that demand careful attention from the scientific and medical communities. In conclusion, the collaboration between AI and neuroscience holds tremendous promise for unraveling the mysteries of the human brain and advancing the understanding of neurological function and dysfunction. By harnessing the capabilities of AI, researchers are forging new pathways towards transformative breakthroughs that have the potential to revolutionize the diagnosis, treatment, and overall comprehension of the intricate workings of the brain.

Ethical Implications of Brain Research

As we delve deeper into the realm of brain research, it becomes increasingly imperative to address the ethical implications that accompany such profound advancements. The intersection of cutting-edge technology and our understanding of the human brain raises significant moral and ethical considerations that must be carefully scrutinized. This section seeks to explore some of the most pressing ethical dilemmas arising from neuroscientific research. One predominant concern relates to the privacy and security of individuals' neural data. With the advent of sophisticated neuroimaging techniques and wearable brain-computer interfaces, questions arise regarding the ownership and potential misuse of this sensitive information. It is essential to establish robust frameworks for data protection and informed consent to ensure that individuals maintain control over their neural data and are safeguarded against exploitation. Additionally, the growing capabilities in neuromodulation raise ethical questions about the potential manipulation of cognitive and emotional states. As researchers gain greater insight into the mechanisms governing brain function, the ethical boundaries of intervention become increasingly pivotal. Striking a balance between therapeutic benefits and respecting individual autonomy is a paramount consideration as we navigate the uncharted territory of brain modulation. Moreover, the use of artificial intelligence (AI) in deciphering complex neural patterns gives rise to ethical quandaries concerning bias and transparency in algorithmic decision-making. Implementing stringent measures to mitigate algorithmic biases and ensuring transparency in AI-driven analyses is crucial to uphold fairness and equity in the interpretation of neuroscientific data. Another critical ethical facet involves the responsible dissemination of neuroscientific findings, particularly in the realms of mental health and cognition. It is vital to prevent the stigmatization of individuals based on neurological characteristics and to foster an environment of empathy and understanding. Ethical guidelines should be established to govern the portrayal and communication of neurological research outcomes, promoting societal inclusivity and eradicating harmful misconceptions. Ultimately, addressing these ethical dimensions necessitates interdisciplinary collaboration and ongoing dialogue among neuroscientists, ethicists, policymakers, and members of the public. By fostering ethical awareness and aligning research endeavors with humanitarian principles, we can strive to harness the immense potential of brain research while upholding the dignity and rights of every individual.

Conclusion: Bridging Knowledge to Practice

In this final section, we have delved deep into the intricate web of ethical considerations that underpin the field of brain research. As we ponder the ethical implications of the advancements in neuroscience and the exploration of the human brain, it becomes evident that an ethical framework is fundamental to guide the progress that science and technology can bring. We have examined the responsibility that comes with wielding knowledge of the brain's inner workings, and the potential impact on individuals and society as a whole. It is crucial for the scientific community, policymakers, and society at large to actively engage in conversations about the ethical boundaries that must be respected. This dialogue must not remain confined within academic circles; it should permeate through every stratum of society. By doing so, we can ensure that the fruits of brain research are harnessed responsibly and ethically. How do we bridge the gap between the knowledge uncovered through research and its practical application in everyday life? This question lies at the heart of the conclusion. The translation of cutting-edge research findings into tangible benefits for individuals facing neurological challenges demands concerted effort from various stakeholders. Clinicians, researchers, and healthcare professionals must collaborate seamlessly to integrate the latest findings into clinical practice. Furthermore, educators and advocates play a vital role in disseminating this knowledge to the wider public sphere, empowering individuals to make informed decisions about brain health. Bridging knowledge to practice also involves addressing systemic barriers, such as access to resources and disparities in healthcare. Advocacy for equitable distribution of resources and support for marginalized communities is essential to ensure that no one is left behind in the journey towards optimal brain health. As we strive to bridge the gap between knowledge and practice, fostering a culture of inclusivity and empathy is paramount. Every individual, irrespective of their background or circumstances, should have the opportunity to benefit from advancements in brain research. In closing, let us recognize that the journey does not end here. The pursuit of understanding the brain and harnessing this knowledge for the betterment of humanity is an ongoing endeavor. It requires continuous collaboration, ethical reflection, and a steadfast commitment to translating knowledge into action. May our shared efforts lead to a future where every individual can realize their full potential, unencumbered by the constraints of brain-related afflictions.

Case Studies or Personal Stories

Introduction to Personal Perspectives

Understanding the personal impact of brain health is an integral part of our journey toward overall well-being. Taking a closer look at personal perspectives allows us to connect with real stories, genuine experiences, and heartfelt triumphs that have the power to inspire and educate. The human brain is at the core of our existence, shaping our thoughts, emotions, and actions. When we delve into personal perspectives, we gain insight into the profound impact that brain health has on individual lives. Each story serves as a testament to resilience, courage, and the unyielding human spirit. By exploring these personal narratives, we uncover the complexities of the brain's influence on our daily lives, relationships, and aspirations. It's within these unique experiences that we find the raw authenticity of human existence, compelling us to appreciate the interconnectedness of mental, emotional, and physical well-being. As we embrace personal perspectives, we open ourselves to empathy, understanding, and a deeper appreciation for the significance of nurturing and maintaining brain health. Through these intimate accounts, we come to recognize the profound and lasting effects of promoting positive brain health and the immeasurable value it holds in enhancing the quality of our lives. Let us embark on this enlightening journey through personal perspectives, where we are invited to embrace the vulnerabilities and strengths encapsulated within each unique story, allowing them to resonate within our own consciousness and inspire meaningful change.

The Story of Jane: Triumph Over Adversity

Jane's journey is a remarkable tale of resilience and triumph over seemingly insurmountable odds. Born into challenging circumstances, she faced numerous obstacles from an early age. Despite the hardships, Jane never lost her courage or determination. Her story is one of unwavering perseverance and unwavering hope. As a young adult, Jane encountered a life-altering event that tested her strength and resolve. Rather than succumbing to despair, she found within herself the fortitude to rise above the adversity. Her unwavering spirit and unyielding faith became the guiding forces in her life. Throughout her journey, Jane's experiences have inspired countless individuals facing their own trials and tribulations. Her willingness to share her story openly and honestly has touched the hearts of many, serving as a beacon of light for those navigating dark and tumultuous paths. Through her unparalleled resilience and steadfast optimism, Jane's narrative serves as a testament to the extraordinary power of the human spirit. Her ability to not only endure, but to flourish in the face of adversity, offers profound insights and invaluable lessons. Jane's story exemplifies the indomitable nature of the human will and illuminates the transformative potential that resides within each and every one of us.

Mark's Journey: Embracing Change

Mark's journey towards embracing change was not an easy one. It began with a sense of uncertainty and fear, as he faced challenges that seemed insurmountable. At the crossroads of his life, Mark realized that change was both inevitable and essential for growth. His story is not just a narrative of personal transformation, but a testament to the resilience of the human spirit. In his early years, Mark found himself caught in the web of monotony and complacency. The mundane rhythm of daily life offered little room for exploration or fulfillment. However, a series of unexpected events propelled him into unfamiliar territory, where he was forced to confront his deepest fears and insecurities. Instead of succumbing to despair, Mark made a conscious decision to confront his doubts and redefine his path forward. Embracing change was not a swift process for Mark. It involved a gradual shift in mindset and a willingness to step outside his comfort zone. He sought guidance from mentors and drew inspiration from individuals who had navigated similar challenges. With each small victory, he gained confidence and momentum, steadily progressing towards a new chapter in his life. The most remarkable aspect of Mark's journey was his ability to embrace vulnerability. He recognized that true strength lies in acknowledging one's weaknesses and leveraging them as catalysts for growth. By allowing himself to be vulnerable, he discovered an unyielding reservoir of courage within him, enabling him to confront adversity with newfound fortitude. As Mark's story unfolds, it becomes evident that change is not merely about altering external circumstances; it is a profound internal shift. He delved into introspection, reevaluating his core values and aspirations. Through this introspective journey, Mark unearthed a reservoir of untapped potential, revealing facets of his personality that had long remained dormant. Mark's journey also serves as a reminder that change is not a solitary endeavor. He found unwavering support from friends, family, and a network of like-minded individuals who propelled him forward during moments of doubt. Their encouragement instilled in him a renewed sense of purpose and accountability, reinforcing his commitment to embracing change. Ultimately, Mark's journey culminated in a transformative metamorphosis, transcending the confines of his initial apprehensions. He emerged as a beacon of hope and inspiration, demonstrating that while change may present formidable obstacles, it also harbors unparalleled opportunities for personal evolution. Mark's journey is a testament to the power of resilience, determination, and the profound rewards that await those who dare to embrace change.

A Mother's Wisdom: Lessons from Experience

It is often said that mothers possess a unique wisdom, forged by the experiences and challenges of raising their children. In this chapter, we delve into the stories of remarkable mothers whose insights have proven invaluable in understanding the complexities of caring for a loved one with neurological struggles. These women have faced adversity with resilience, compassion, and unwavering dedication.

Through their narratives, we gain profound lessons that transcend the pages of any book or academic discourse. One such mother is Sarah, whose son Ben was diagnosed with a rare neurological condition at a young age. Despite the uncertainty and fear that clouded her world, Sarah approached her son's care with an unparalleled sense of strength and determination. She learned to navigate the labyrinthine healthcare system, became an advocate for her son, and found solace in connecting with other parents facing similar challenges. Her tenacity and relentless pursuit of knowledge not only transformed Ben's life but also inspired countless others on similar paths. From Sarah's story, we learn the importance of resilience and the immeasurable impact of a mother's love. Another remarkable figure is Maria, whose daughter Ava was born with a congenital neurological condition. Maria's unwavering devotion to Ava's well-being led her on a journey of discovery, pushing the boundaries of traditional medicine in search of holistic therapies and alternative treatments. Her tireless efforts not only improved Ava's quality of life but also ignited hope within a community grappling with similar circumstances. Maria's story serves as a testament to the power of maternal intuition and the boundless determination to explore every avenue for the benefit of a child. These exemplary mothers illuminate the path forward for others navigating the daunting terrain of neurological care. Their profound insights teach us the value of unconditional love, the significance of empowerment through advocacy, and the transformative influence of hope. As we immerse ourselves in their experiences, we are reminded that amidst the scientific studies and medical analyses, it is often the wisdom and resilience of these mothers that provide the greatest guidance and comfort in the realm of neurological care.

Community Support: The Power of Togetherness

In exploring the profound impact of community support, it becomes evident that the power of togetherness cannot be overstated. From organized support groups to informal networks of care, communities play a pivotal role in providing comfort, guidance, and strength to individuals facing neurological challenges. The sense of belonging and understanding that arises from shared experiences is invaluable, fostering a deep sense of empathy and solidarity among members. Through mutual encouragement and shared resources, communities serve as a vital lifeline for those navigating the complexities of neurological conditions. It is within these communities that individuals not only find solace but also practical assistance. Whether through emotional reassurance, knowledge exchange, or tangible aid, the collective effort of a community can alleviate the burden carried by individuals and their caregivers. This collaborative approach contributes to a nurturing environment where every voice is heard, valued, and supported. Such cohesion fosters an environment where hope flourishes, and individuals feel empowered to face their struggles with resilience and optimism. Moreover, the impact of community support extends beyond the individual level, influencing societal perceptions and driving positive change. By raising awareness and advocating for improved services and resources, communities exemplify the strength derived from unity in confronting neurological challenges. Embracing inclusivity and diversity, these communal endeavors promote empathy, understanding, and equitable treatment for all. Through the symbiotic relationship between individuals and their communities, a culture of support and compassion emerges, ultimately shaping a more compassionate and informed society. As we continue to recognize and harness the transformative influence of community support, it becomes evident that together, we are capable of overcoming obstacles and advancing towards a future of shared prosperity and well-being.

Learning from the Past: Historical Case Studies

Throughout history, individuals and communities have faced various neurological and cognitive challenges. Examining these historical case studies not only provides valuable insight into the progression of our understanding of the brain but also offers inspiration and guidance for those currently navigating similar experiences. One notable historical case is that of Phineas Gage, a railroad construction foreman who, in 1848, survived a traumatic brain injury that dramatically altered his personality and behavior. Gage's case provided critical early evidence of the brain's role in regulating emotions and social interactions, shaping the foundation of modern neurology and psychology. Another compelling example is the life of Henrietta Lacks, whose unique cells, taken without her consent in 1951, formed the first immortal human cell line, contributing significantly to scientific research on various medical conditions, including brain-related disorders. Exploring these cases allows us to appreciate the resilience and adaptability of individuals, as well as the crucial role of these narratives in advancing medical knowledge. As we consider these historical accounts, we must acknowledge the ethical considerations surrounding them and honor the individuals who have contributed, often unknowingly, to the advancement of neuroscience. By learning from the stories of those who came before us, we gain a deeper understanding of the complexities of the human brain and a renewed appreciation for the progress we have made in our approach to brain health and care.

Voices of Experts: Insights from the Field

In this section, we have the privilege of delving into the invaluable insights shared by experts in the field of neuroscience and psychology. Through their dedicated work, these professionals have contributed to our understanding of the human brain and its remarkable capabilities. As we immerse ourselves in their knowledge and experience, we gain a deeper appreciation for the intricate workings of the mind. The voices of these experts resonate with passion and wisdom, offering us a window into the evolving landscape of brain research. From neuroscientists exploring the frontiers of cognitive function to psychologists unraveling the complexities of behavior, each expert provides a unique perspective that enriches our exploration of the human brain. Their collective wisdom not only informs our understanding of the past but also illuminates the path forward, guiding us toward better strategies for nurturing mental well-being. Through their insights, we are reminded of the immense potential for growth and resilience within each individual. Furthermore, the experts remind us of the importance of interdisciplinary collaboration in advancing our understanding of the brain, emphasizing the need for holistic approaches that consider both biological and psychological factors. Their dedication to sharing knowledge and enhancing public awareness inspires us to continue seeking innovative solutions for addressing neurological challenges and promoting mental wellness. As we absorb the wealth of information they provide, we are encouraged to apply these insights to our everyday lives, fostering an environment that supports cognitive health and emotional flourishing. The voices of these experts serve as beacons of inspiration, instilling confidence in our collective ability to shape a future where the limitless potential of the human brain is celebrated and safeguarded.

Facing the Future: Stories of Hope

In this section, we delve into the inspiring stories of individuals who have overcome tremendous challenges and emerged stronger, offering hope and encouragement to others facing similar struggles. These narratives showcase the resilience of the human spirit and the transformative power of perseverance. One such story is that of Maria, a young woman who battled a debilitating illness for years. Despite numerous setbacks, Maria never lost sight of her dreams and aspirations. Through unwavering determination and the unwavering support of her loved ones, she not only conquered her illness but also went on to pursue her passion for helping others in need. Her journey serves as a testament to the triumph of hope over adversity. Similarly, we are introduced to the remarkable journey of David, a war veteran who faced immense physical and emotional trauma. Through his unwavering resolve and with the aid of innovative medical treatments, David not only regained his physical abilities but also dedicated his life to supporting fellow veterans and advocating for mental health awareness. His story exemplifies the indomitable strength of the human will. We also encounter the touching account of Sarah, a single mother who defied all odds to provide a better future for her children. Despite financial hardships and societal challenges, Sarah's resilience and resourcefulness enabled her to create opportunities for her family, inspiring others in similar circumstances to strive for a brighter tomorrow. These narratives of hope and resilience do more than inspire—they illuminate the path forward for those grappling with their own obstacles. They offer insight, motivation, and a profound reminder that adversity can be the catalyst for remarkable personal growth. The unique experiences shared within these stories remind us that no matter how daunting the circumstances, there is always a way to navigate through the storm and emerge stronger on the other side. The tales of these courageous individuals serve as guiding lights, affirming that a brighter future is within reach for all those who dare to believe.

Lessons Learned: Reflective Thoughts

In this chapter, we have delved into the intimate and inspiring stories of individuals who have faced significant challenges, yet emerged victorious through resilience, determination, and unwavering hope. As we reflect on these stories, it is undeniable that they impart invaluable lessons that resonate across time and circumstances. One recurring theme in these personal narratives is the power of the human spirit to triumph over adversity. The reflections of individuals like Jane, Mark, and numerous others serve as profound reminders of the resilience inherent within us all. Their experiences underscore the potential for growth and transformation, even in the face of seemingly insurmountable obstacles. Their stories motivate us to embrace change and approach life's challenges with courage and optimism. Furthermore, these personal anecdotes shed light on the significance of community support and empathy. Whether it is the unwavering love of a devoted mother or the solidarity found in shared experiences, these narratives emphasize the pivotal role of social connections in navigating difficult times. They underscore the profound impact of compassion, understanding, and unity in fostering hope and healing. Moreover, the historical case studies included in this chapter offer timeless wisdom and insights. By examining the journeys of individuals from generations past, we gain a deeper appreciation for the enduring nature of human resilience. These stories serve as beacons of wisdom, illuminating the path forward and providing valuable perspective on the universal nature of the human experience. As we pause to contemplate the reflective thoughts elicited by these poignant narratives, it becomes evident that embracing the lessons learned from these stories is essential. Through introspection and contemplation, we can internalize the wisdom distilled from these experiences. We are reminded of the profound impact of hope, determination, and community in shaping our lives and guiding our paths forward. Ultimately, the lessons gleaned from these personal stories are not merely isolated accounts, but rather, they represent universal truths that resonate deeply within the human experience. They inspire us to embark on our own journeys of self-discovery, growth, and compassionate connection with those around us.

The Next Steps: Bridging to Practical Care

After reflecting on the profound experiences shared in the previous chapters, it becomes evident that true understanding leads to action. As we embrace the valuable lessons learned from these personal stories and case studies, it is essential to consider how we can translate this knowledge into actionable steps for practical care. The journey of caregiving or self-care often requires a thoughtful approach that integrates both empathy and practicality. This section aims to explore the next steps in bridging the inspirational narratives we've encountered with meaningful and tangible care practices. First and foremost, it's crucial to recognize that every individual's situation is unique. The nuances and complexities of each story underscore the importance of tailoring care to specific needs. The next step involves gaining a comprehensive understanding of the available resources and support systems. From community organizations to medical professionals, tapping into these networks can provide invaluable guidance and assistance in navigating the challenges associated with brain health and wellness. Furthermore, building on the reflective thoughts derived from personal stories, it's time to delve into the development of proactive strategies for sustainable care. This may involve creating personalized care plans, integrating therapeutic activities, or exploring innovative technologies designed to enhance cognitive function. The significance of taking practical steps cannot be overstated, as they serve as the bedrock for impactful and enduring care journeys. In addition to personalized strategies, the next steps must also encompass the vital aspect of education and awareness. Empowering individuals with knowledge about brain health and caregiving best practices is fundamental in fostering a supportive environment. By disseminating information through workshops, seminars, and educational materials, we can collectively contribute to a community-wide culture of understanding and proactive engagement. Finally, the next steps involve advocating for sustained support systems that prioritize the holistic well-being of individuals and families impacted by brain-related challenges. Whether through policy initiatives or grassroots efforts, amplifying voices and championing inclusive care initiatives are pivotal in fostering an environment where compassion and practical care intersect. As we embark on this journey towards practical care, let the narratives we've encountered serve as guiding lights, illuminating the path towards meaningful and impactful actions. The next steps are not only about implementing strategies but also about fostering a community ethos rooted in empathy, understanding, and unwavering support. Together, we can bridge the personal stories to real-world care, making a difference in the lives of those navigating the intricate landscape of brain health and wellness.

Practical Tips for Everyday Care

Introduction to Everyday Care

As we embark on the journey of caring for our well-being, it is crucial to understand that each individual has distinct needs and requirements when it comes to achieving optimal health. Understanding your unique needs involves delving into the specific factors that contribute to your physical, mental, and emotional balance. Factors such as age, genetics, lifestyle, and any existing health conditions play a pivotal role in shaping your personal care routine. By recognizing and acknowledging these individual aspects, you can tailor your approach towards self-care to resonate with your body's innate requirements. It's important to remember that what works for one person may not necessarily yield the same results for another. Therefore, taking the time to identify and comprehend your unique needs is the cornerstone of establishing an effective and sustainable daily care regimen.

Understanding Your Unique Needs

Understanding your unique needs is a pivotal aspect of caring for your brain health. Each individual possesses a distinct set of requirements, influenced by genetic predispositions, lifestyle choices, and environmental factors. At the core of understanding your unique needs lies the recognition that no two people are exactly alike, and therefore, a personalized approach to care is essential. It begins with a deep introspection into your own habits, preferences, and challenges. Assessing your current state of mental and physical well-being can provide valuable insights into areas that require attention and improvement. This process also involves acknowledging the impact of external influences on your brain health. Consider the demands of your work, family dynamics, social interactions, and community involvement. Reflect on how these aspects influence your stress levels, cognitive functioning, and emotional resilience. By recognizing the interconnectedness of these factors with your brain health, you can gain a clearer understanding of the specific care regimen that will best support your overall well-being. Furthermore, embracing an understanding of your unique needs entails engaging in conversations with healthcare professionals, seeking their guidance, and leveraging their expertise. Collaborating with medical practitioners, nutritionists, fitness trainers, and mental health counselors can provide invaluable direction in customizing your care plan. Through open and honest discussions, you can gain deeper insights into your body's requirements and how to fulfill them optimally. In addition to seeking external expertise, self-awareness plays a vital role in this journey. Taking the time for mindful reflection and self-evaluation can reveal patterns, triggers, and areas of strength that are crucial in tailoring your approach to brain health. It is essential to approach this process with compassion and patience, recognizing that meaningful change takes time and effort. Embracing your uniqueness and integrating it into your care routine can foster a sense of empowerment and autonomy, leading to a more fulfilling and effective health maintenance strategy. Ultimately, understanding your unique needs sets the foundation for a holistic and sustainable approach to brain health. Honoring your individuality while proactively addressing your specific requirements empowers you to make informed decisions and prioritizes self-care. With this knowledge, you can confidently progress towards optimizing your brain health and enhancing your overall quality of life.

Building a Daily Routine

The foundation of holistic well-being lies in the cultivation of a balanced and nurturing daily routine. Establishing a predictable schedule can significantly enhance your overall health and cognitive function. Begin by setting consistent waking and sleeping times to regulate your body's internal clock, aiming for seven to eight hours of high-quality sleep each night. This helps optimize brain function and emotional stability, offering the essential restoration needed for mental sharpness and resilience throughout the day. Additionally, incorporating regular meal times into your daily regimen nurtures both physical and mental vitality. Fueling your body with wholesome, nutritious foods at consistent intervals maintains stable blood sugar levels, sustaining energy and concentration. Moreover, by integrating short breaks for movement or relaxation, you can refresh your mind and alleviate the strain of prolonged mental exertion. Consider engaging in mindfulness practices, such as meditation or deep breathing exercises, to promote emotional balance and reduce stress. Furthermore, allotting time for leisure activities that bring you joy and fulfillment fosters psychological well-being. Whether it's reading, creative expression, or socializing, these pursuits contribute to a balanced and harmonious life. Crafting a daily routine tailored to your specific needs and aspirations empowers you to lead a purposeful and fulfilling existence, where your brain and body thrive in harmony.

Mindful Eating Habits

Mindful eating is a practice that encourages individuals to pay full attention to the experience of eating, from the selection and preparation of food to the actual consumption. It involves being present in the moment and engaging all the senses to truly savor and appreciate the nourishment we receive from food. This section will delve into the importance of mindful eating habits and how they can positively impact overall well-being. In today's fast-paced world, it's easy to fall into the habit of mindless or distracted eating. Many of us have experienced moments when we've rushed through a meal while working at our desks, watching television, or scrolling through our phones. However, this can lead to overeating or not fully appreciating the food we consume. Mindful eating offers an alternative approach by encouraging individuals to slow down and be fully present during meals. One fundamental aspect of mindful eating is developing a deeper awareness of hunger and satiety cues. By tuning into our body's signals, we can better understand when we are truly hungry versus experiencing emotional or habitual cravings. Additionally, mindful eating emphasizes the need to cultivate a more profound connection with the food we eat. This involves considering the sources of our food, acknowledging the effort involved in its production, and expressing gratitude for the nourishment it provides. Furthermore, practicing mindfulness during meals allows individuals to appreciate the sensory aspects of eating. It involves observing the colors, textures, aromas, and flavors of the food on our plate. Engaging all the senses in this way enhances the dining experience and fosters a greater sense of satisfaction from our meals. Through mindful eating, individuals can cultivate a healthier relationship with food, leading to improved digestion, reduced stress, and an overall enhanced appreciation for nourishment. Incorporating mindful eating habits into daily life requires patience and practice. It's essential to start with small steps, such as taking a few deep breaths before a meal to center yourself, chewing slowly and thoroughly, and setting aside distractions while eating. Over time, these practices can become ingrained habits that promote a healthier and more fulfilling relationship with food. By embracing mindful eating, individuals can enrich their lives and well-being, one bite at a time.

The Importance of Sleep

Sleep is an essential component of overall well-being and plays a crucial role in maintaining a healthy brain. In today's fast-paced world, it's easy to underestimate the importance of quality sleep, often prioritizing work, social activities, or other obligations. However, the significance of sufficient and restorative sleep cannot be overstated. When we sleep, our bodies and brains undergo a series of vital processes that contribute to our physical and mental health. From consolidating memories to repairing tissue and regulating hormones, sleep is the cornerstone of our body's recovery and rejuvenation. Furthermore, adequate sleep is directly linked to enhanced cognitive function, emotional regulation, and overall productivity. Many studies have shown that individuals who consistently obtain the recommended amount of sleep report higher levels of focus, creativity, and problem-solving abilities. Moreover, a well-rested mind is better equipped to handle stress and maintain a positive outlook on life. On the contrary, chronic sleep deprivation has been associated with a myriad of negative consequences, including increased risk of developing various health conditions, impaired immune function, and heightened susceptibility to mood disorders. It's important to recognize that the quality of sleep is just as crucial as the quantity. Creating a conducive sleep environment, adhering to a regular sleep schedule, and practicing relaxation techniques can significantly improve the depth and restfulness of your sleep. As you embark on your journey to prioritize sleep, keep in mind that achieving optimal sleep habits requires mindfulness and dedication. By acknowledging the pivotal role of sleep in our overall health and making proactive choices to support it, we can cultivate a more vibrant and fulfilling life.

Incorporating Physical Activity

Physical activity is an essential component of overall well-being, playing a crucial role in maintaining a healthy mind and body. The benefits of regular exercise are far-reaching and encompass various aspects of our health. Engaging in physical activity not only improves cardiovascular health and muscle strength but also enhances mental clarity and emotional resilience. It's important to understand that physical activity doesn't have to be intense or time-consuming to be beneficial. Incorporating simple activities into your daily routine can make a significant difference. Whether it's taking a brisk walk, practicing yoga, swimming, or dancing, finding activities that you enjoy is key to making physical activity a sustainable part of your life. Regular movement has been shown to reduce the risk of chronic diseases such as heart disease, diabetes, and obesity. It also promotes better sleep, boosts energy levels, and helps manage weight effectively. Furthermore, engaging in physical activity releases endorphins, which are natural stress-relievers and mood-boosters. This can contribute to a more positive outlook on life and increased overall satisfaction. In addition to the physical benefits, incorporating regular physical activity into your life can also help build discipline, self-confidence, and a sense of achievement. It provides an opportunity for self-care and introspection, allowing you to disconnect from the stresses of daily life and focus on your personal well-being. When implementing physical activity into your routine, start with small, manageable goals and gradually increase intensity and duration as your fitness improves. Remember that consistency is key, and even short bursts of activity throughout the day can add up to significant health benefits. By making physical activity a priority, you're investing in your present and future health. As you embrace the power of movement, you'll discover the transformative impact it can have on your overall wellness and quality of life.

Managing Stress Effectively

Life can be filled with various stressors, from work demands and financial responsibilities to personal relationships and unexpected challenges. It's essential to recognize the impact that stress can have on our overall well-being, both physically and mentally. Managing stress effectively is not only crucial for maintaining good mental health but also for promoting a harmonious and balanced lifestyle. One effective way to manage stress is by incorporating relaxation techniques into our daily routines. Engaging in activities such as meditation, deep breathing exercises, or yoga can help calm the mind and reduce the physiological symptoms of stress. Additionally, finding healthy outlets for stress, such as engaging in hobbies or spending time in nature, can provide a much-needed mental break. Another vital aspect of stress management is maintaining a strong support system. Whether it's through close friends, family members, or professional counseling, having a network of individuals who can provide emotional support and guidance can significantly alleviate stress. Additionally, practicing mindful awareness and staying present in the current moment can prevent unnecessary worry about the future and regret about the past. Developing healthy coping mechanisms, such as maintaining a positive attitude and finding gratitude in everyday moments, can also contribute to effective stress management. Moreover, setting realistic goals and boundaries, both in personal and professional spheres, can help reduce overwhelming feelings of stress. Finally, it's important to remember that seeking help is not a sign of weakness but an act of self-care. If stress becomes overwhelming and begins to interfere with daily life, seeking professional help from a therapist or counselor is a proactive step towards managing stress effectively. By implementing these strategies and recognizing the significance of stress management, individuals can cultivate resilience and improve their overall well-being.

Nurturing Mental Health

In the pursuit of overall well-being, it is imperative to not overlook the significance of nurturing our mental health. Our emotions, thoughts, and behaviors are all interconnected with our mental state, making it an essential aspect of our holistic wellness. Nurturing mental health involves acknowledging and managing our emotions, fostering a positive mindset, and seeking support when needed. Embracing mindfulness and self-compassion can significantly contribute to strengthening our mental resilience. One fundamental element in nurturing mental health is understanding the impact of stress on our psychological well-being. Chronic stress can take a toll on mental health, leading to anxiety, depression, and other adverse effects. Therefore, implementing stress management techniques, such as meditation, deep breathing exercises, and engaging in activities that bring joy and relaxation, is pivotal in safeguarding our mental equilibrium. Moreover, fostering meaningful connections and cultivating a strong support system play a vital role in nurturing mental health. Social interactions, empathy, and open communication offer a platform for sharing experiences and seeking comfort during challenging times. Actively participating in social activities and surrounding ourselves with individuals who uplift and encourage us can profoundly impact our mental well-being. Self-care practices also form an integral part of nurturing mental health. Engaging in activities that bring joy, practicing gratitude, and setting aside time for hobbies and interests contribute to a sense of fulfillment and contentment. Additionally, prioritizing adequate rest and relaxation is paramount in preserving mental clarity and emotional stability. Understanding and addressing mental health concerns without stigma or judgment is crucial. Seeking professional support from therapists, counselors, or mental health professionals should be considered a courageous step towards nurturing one's mental well-being. It signifies strength and self-awareness in recognizing the need for guidance and intervention. Lastly, promoting mental health awareness within our communities and workplaces fosters an environment of empathy and understanding. Initiating conversations about mental health, advocating for resources and support, and dispelling myths and stereotypes contribute to creating a more inclusive and supportive atmosphere for everyone. In essence, nurturing mental health requires a holistic approach that encompasses self-awareness, self-compassion, and proactive engagement with various aspects of our lives. It empowers us to embrace challenges with resilience and navigate through complexities with a strengthened mental fortitude.

Staying Informed About Your Health

As we navigate the complexities of modern life, staying informed about our health is a crucial cornerstone of overall well-being. The world of healthcare and wellness is constantly evolving, with new research, treatments, and insights emerging regularly. Therefore, it's essential for individuals to take an active role in understanding and staying updated about their health. This involves fostering an ongoing relationship with healthcare providers, engaging in regular health screenings and check-ups, and remaining curious and inquisitive about personal health matters. By keeping abreast of the latest medical developments and maintaining open communication with healthcare professionals, individuals can make more informed decisions about their health and treatment options. Moreover, staying informed also empowers individuals to recognize potential warning signs or symptoms early on, leading to timely interventions and improved outcomes. However, it's equally important to approach health information critically, distinguishing between reliable sources and misinformation. Developing sound research skills and seeking guidance from reputable healthcare professionals can help individuals separate facts from myths, enabling them to make well-informed choices. Embracing lifelong learning about health not only enhances personal well-being but also fosters a proactive approach to self-care. Whether through reading reputable health publications, attending educational workshops, or participating in community health initiatives, staying informed becomes a continual journey toward better health. Beyond personal benefits, this knowledge-sharing ethos within communities can contribute to a collective culture of wellness, promoting healthier and more informed societies. Ultimately, staying informed about health is an empowering and proactive endeavor that paves the way for individuals to lead healthier, more fulfilling lives.

Embracing Positivity and Gratitude

In the journey towards holistic well-being, cultivating positivity and gratitude can play a profound role in shaping our mental and emotional landscape. Embracing a positive mindset involves acknowledging challenges while consciously choosing to focus on the bright spots amidst the complexities of life. It's about nurturing an optimistic outlook that propels us forward, even in the face of adversity. Practicing gratitude, on the other hand, encourages us to recognize and appreciate the blessings, big and small, that enrich our lives. It empowers us to shift our attention to the abundance that surrounds us, fostering a profound sense of contentment and fulfillment. The practice of embracing positivity and gratitude is intertwined with our overall health and well-being. Research has shown that individuals who adopt a positive mindset exhibit lower levels of stress and anxiety, contributing to improved mental and emotional resilience. By fostering gratitude, we not only enhance our psychological state but also bolster our physical health by reducing inflammation and promoting better sleep patterns. Cultivating these qualities has been found to enhance overall life satisfaction and increase levels of optimism, ultimately fortifying our psychological immune system against life's inevitable ups and downs. Furthermore, integrating positivity and gratitude into daily life involves a conscious effort to reframe our perspectives. This may involve daily affirmations, mindfulness practices, or engaging in acts of kindness towards others. Pausing to savor the present moment, reflecting on moments of joy, and expressing appreciation for the people and experiences that enrich our lives can significantly contribute to a more positive and grateful outlook. Engaging in activities like journaling about uplifting experiences, volunteering, or simply taking a moment to connect with nature can serve as powerful reminders of the abundance in our lives. Ultimately, embracing positivity and gratitude is not about dismissing challenges or hardships but rather about acknowledging them while actively seeking the silver linings and finding reasons to be grateful. By infusing our lives with positivity and gratitude, we open ourselves to a world of possibilities, resilience, and inner peace. It becomes a transformative practice that amplifies our capacity for joy, resilience, and empathy, enriching our lives and radiating positivity to those around us. As we navigate the complexities of modern living, fostering these traits becomes a beacon of hope, guiding us towards a more fulfilling and rewarding existence.

Disclaimer

Purpose of the Disclaimer

The purpose of including this disclaimer in the book is to ensure that readers understand the guidelines and limitations surrounding the information provided. It serves as a means of setting clear expectations and delineating the boundaries of the knowledge shared within these pages. By acknowledging the importance of this disclaimer, readers can approach the content with mindfulness and discernment, recognizing that while it offers valuable insights, it cannot replace individualized professional advice. In doing so, the aim is to promote a responsible and informed engagement with the material, fostering a sense of awareness about the scope and boundaries of the information presented. Ultimately, the intent of this disclaimer is to encourage readers to approach the forthcoming chapters with a balanced perspective, utilizing the knowledge gained as a complement to, rather than a substitute for, personalized guidance from qualified professionals.

General Information and Advice

In this section, we aim to provide comprehensive insights into the general information and advice related to brain health without being a substitute for professional guidance. It is crucial to understand that while our intention is to offer valuable knowledge, every individual's healthcare concerns and conditions are unique. The content presented here serves as a springboard for further exploration and learning about maintaining brain health. Always prioritize consulting with qualified healthcare professionals for personalized advice and treatment. With that said, it's important to acknowledge that general information and advice can significantly contribute to promoting overall well-being. By understanding the basic principles of brain functioning, individuals can make informed decisions and incorporate positive lifestyle changes. Whether it's the significance of nutrition, exercise, or mental stimulation, this section delves into the fundamental aspects that play a key role in optimizing brain health. We encourage readers to approach this information with an open mind, considering it a starting point for a deeper understanding of holistic well-being. It is our sincere hope that by providing general information and advice, readers will be empowered to take proactive steps towards nurturing their cognitive abilities and achieving a balanced and fulfilling life. Furthermore, recognizing the importance of regular check-ups and preventative measures cannot be overstated. Together, let us embark on a journey of discovery, embracing the value of knowledge and the pursuit of optimal brain health.

Not a Substitute for Professional Guidance

This book is intended to provide valuable information and insights into the complexities of brain health. However, it is important to emphasize that the content presented within these pages is not a substitute for professional guidance from qualified medical and healthcare professionals. While the aim is to empower readers with knowledge and practical advice, it is crucial to recognize the limitations of self-help resources in addressing individual health concerns. The human brain is a remarkably intricate organ, and its functions can vary widely from person to person. As such, it is imperative to acknowledge the necessity of personalized, professional care when dealing with any neurological or cognitive issues. Acknowledging this fact is not a sign of weakness, but rather an indication of prudence and a commitment to one's well-being. Seeking professional guidance ensures access to tailored assessments, accurate diagnoses, and comprehensive treatment plans that consider the full spectrum of an individual's health needs. This is especially essential given the rapidly evolving nature of medical knowledge and interventions. While this book endeavors to offer educational value, it cannot replace the expertise provided by trained specialists who have devoted their careers to understanding and addressing brain-related conditions. Readers are urged to engage with healthcare professionals and participate actively in conversations about their cognitive and neurological health. Likewise, family members and caregivers are encouraged to support and advocate for their loved ones in seeking expert assistance when necessary. By fostering open dialogue and partnerships with healthcare providers, individuals can avail themselves of the best possible care and guidance. Furthermore, in cases of emergency or acute health concerns, prompt access to professional medical attention is indispensable. Understanding the distinction between informative resources and professional medical advice is vital in making informed decisions about one's well-being. This delineation serves as a cornerstone in maintaining a balanced and responsible approach to brain health. As we navigate through the intricacies of understanding and nurturing our minds, let us do so with an unwavering commitment to integrating professional guidance into our personal journeys toward optimal brain health.

Limitations of This Book's Content

Readers, it is essential to understand the boundaries and constraints that come with the content presented in this book. While every effort has been made to assemble accurate and up-to-date information, it is crucial to acknowledge the inherent limitations. The field of neuroscience and brain health is dynamic, continuously evolving alongside advancements in scientific research and medical practice. As such, this book may not capture the very latest developments or encompass the entirety of the vast knowledge within this domain. It is essential for readers to recognize that the material presented here is a distillation of complex topics and should be viewed as a starting point rather than a comprehensive resource. Furthermore, individual cases and circumstances vary widely, and while the content aims to be broadly informative, it cannot address every unique situation comprehensively. Each reader's journey towards understanding and caring for their brain health will necessitate additional sources of information and personalized guidance from healthcare professionals. It is also important to note that this book does not constitute personalized medical advice, diagnosis, or treatment. Readers are encouraged to consult with qualified healthcare providers to address their specific needs and concerns. Additionally, the cultural and contextual diversity of individuals globally presents a challenge in creating universally applicable content. While efforts have been made to ensure the inclusivity and relevance of the material, readers are encouraged to consider their unique backgrounds and seek supplementary sources that resonate with their cultural, regional, and personal perspectives. Despite these limitations, the intent behind this book remains steadfast – to empower and equip readers with fundamental knowledge and practical insights into brain health. By emphasizing awareness and encouraging proactive engagement, the aim is to guide readers towards seeking further guidance and enhancing their overall well-being. In recognizing the constraints of this resource, readers can approach its content with a discerning mindset, fostering an ongoing pursuit of knowledge and understanding beyond the scope of this book.

Author's Expertise and Intentions

As the author of this book, it is crucial for me to share with you my expertise and intentions in writing about the complexities of the human brain. My deep-seated passion for neuroscience stems from years of dedicated study and research in this field. Having earned advanced degrees and devoted countless hours to exploring the intricacies of the brain, I bring a wealth of knowledge and experience to the pages of this book. It is my sincerest desire to empower and educate readers about the fascinating workings of the brain, shedding light on its functions and the factors that impact its health and well-being. My intention in crafting this literary piece is not only to impart information but also to cultivate an environment of understanding and compassion. Throughout my career, I have witnessed the profound impact that awareness and insight can have on individuals grappling with neurological challenges. By sharing my expertise through this book, I aim to offer solace, inspiration, and actionable guidance to those navigating the complexities of brain-related issues. This book is a testament to my unyielding commitment to advancing public awareness and understanding of the brain, with the ultimate goal of contributing to improved mental and cognitive well-being for all. It is important for readers to understand that my motivations extend beyond a mere academic or professional pursuit. I am driven by a sincere desire to make a tangible difference in the lives of individuals and communities affected by neurological conditions. Through the dissemination of comprehensive and reliable information, I seek to promote increased empathy, support, and effective interventions within society. My intentions are rooted in the genuine belief that by fostering a deeper comprehension of the brain, we can nurture a more empathetic and inclusive community where individuals facing cognitive health challenges are embraced, supported, and provided with the resources they need to thrive. I want to assure you, as a reader, that the insights and recommendations presented in this book are deeply rooted in scientific rigor and ethical consideration. It is my personal and professional commitment to uphold the highest standards of integrity and accuracy throughout the entirety of this literary endeavor. My expertise and intentions converge to create a narrative that endeavors to uplift and enlighten, offering a foundation of trust and reliability upon which readers can build their own understanding and seek avenues for personal growth and development. As we embark on this enlightening journey together, my hope is that you will find in these pages not only a source of knowledge and guidance but also a testament to the unwavering sincerity and dedication with which this book has been crafted. I stand behind this work as a reflection of my lifelong commitment to advocating for the welfare and understanding of the intricate organ that is the brain. May the chapters ahead resonate with your curiosity, inspire your empathy, and equip you with the tools to navigate the complexities of the brain with confidence and compassion.

Encouragement to Seek Medical Advice

Seeking medical advice is crucial when it comes to your health and well-being. While this book aims to provide valuable insights and practical tips, it's important to acknowledge that every individual has unique physical and mental characteristics that may require personalized attention from medical professionals. Protecting your health means being proactive and informed, and consulting with a healthcare provider can offer you tailored guidance suited to your specific needs. Whether you are considering making significant lifestyle changes, embarking on a new exercise routine, or altering your diet, the input of a qualified medical professional can help ensure that you make choices that align with your best interests. Moreover, in cases where you have existing medical conditions or are taking medications, professional advice can prevent potential contraindications or complications. It's essential to recognize that no general information or advice, no matter how thoughtfully presented, can replace the individualized care and assessment provided by a licensed physician or healthcare practitioner. Your health is too valuable to leave to mere chance or speculation. By actively involving medical experts in your health-related decisions, you demonstrate a commitment to safeguarding your overall wellness and gaining peace of mind. In doing so, you empower yourself to make informed choices while benefiting from the expertise and experience of those dedicated to advancing and preserving your health and longevity.

Liability and Responsibility

In producing this book, our utmost priority is to provide accurate and reliable information about the brain and its functions. However, it's crucial to recognize the limitations and nuances associated with medical and scientific literature. The content shared in this book is intended for informational purposes only, and while every effort has been made to ensure its accuracy, we cannot guarantee that all the information provided is current, complete, or applicable to every individual's circumstances. As a reader, it's important to understand the inherent risks of self-diagnosis or treatment based solely on the information presented here. We strongly advise that any decisions regarding your health be made in consultation with qualified medical professionals who can offer personalized advice and care tailored to your specific needs. Moreover, as the author, I acknowledge the responsibility that comes with sharing knowledge about such a complex and sensitive topic. While I have drawn upon reputable sources and my own expertise in crafting this book, I must emphasize that its contents are not a replacement for professional medical guidance. Readers should exercise caution and discretion when applying any information from this book to their own situations, and should always seek guidance from certified healthcare providers. It's essential to recognize that individual responses to treatments and lifestyle changes can vary, and what works well for one person may not have the same effect for another. Therefore, the liability for any action taken based on the information in this book rests solely with the reader and their healthcare providers. I, as the author, accept the obligation to continuously review and update this material to reflect the latest developments in relevant fields. However, I cannot assume responsibility for any errors, omissions, or outcomes resulting from the use of this book's content. I encourage readers to approach the information with an open mind, critically assessing its applicability in their unique circumstances. As we progress through this exploration of the brain, it's vital to maintain a balanced perspective, acknowledging the complexities and individuality of each person's medical journey. By recognizing the shared responsibility between the author, the reader, and healthcare professionals, we can foster a more informed and collaborative approach to brain health.

Endorsements and Affiliations

In order to provide you with the most transparent and honest information, it is important to address any endorsements or affiliations that may have influenced the content of this book. I want to assure you that the recommendations and insights shared within these pages are based solely on my genuine belief in their value and potential to benefit your understanding of the brain and its functions. It is essential to clarify that this book does not aim to promote or endorse any specific product, brand, or organization. Any mentioned products or services are purely for illustrative and educational purposes, and do not constitute an endorsement by myself or the publishers. Additionally, any affiliations or relationships with organizations or companies disclosed in this book are purely for transparency and do not impact the objectivity of the information provided. Transparency is paramount when discussing affiliations and associations, so I want to emphasize that while there might be professional connections to certain entities, they have not influenced the content presented. My intention is always to prioritize the readers' best interests and offer unbiased knowledge regarding the brain's intricacies. I understand the importance of maintaining independence and impartiality, which is why every effort has been made to ensure that the information presented is free from any undue influence. This commitment extends to any affiliate links or partnerships that may be referenced, as they are included with full disclosure and solely intended to enrich the reader's experience. Your trust in the authenticity and integrity of the information offered in this book is paramount. As such, I am dedicated to upholding a standard of honesty and forthrightness when it comes to any affiliations or potential influences within the context of this publication. Please feel confident that the content has been curated with the sole purpose of empowering you with valuable insights into the fascinating world of the human brain.

Updates and Revisions

As research and understanding of the brain continue to evolve, it is imperative that this book remains current and reflective of the latest knowledge and insights. Therefore, regular updates and revisions are essential to ensure that readers are presented with accurate, up-to-date information about brain health. Understanding the dynamic nature of scientific progress, the author is committed to diligently reviewing and incorporating any new findings or developments in the field of neuroscience. It is the author's sincere intention to provide readers with the most relevant and reliable information available. In the spirit of transparency and integrity, all revisions and updates will be clearly documented, highlighting the changes made and the reasons behind them. This commitment to ongoing improvement aims to enhance the value and utility of this book for its readers. Additionally, feedback from readers, healthcare professionals, and experts in the field will be actively welcomed and considered when making updates and revisions. This collaborative approach ensures that diverse perspectives and expertise contribute to the continual enhancement of this resource. As a result, readers can trust that this book is a dynamic, living document that adapts to reflect the latest advancements and discoveries in brain science. The importance of staying informed and educated about brain health cannot be overstated, and the author remains dedicated to ensuring that this book fulfills its role as an authoritative and informative guide. By staying true to the commitment of updates and revisions, this book aims to empower readers with the most current and credible knowledge about the intricate workings of the human brain.

Final Words Before Moving Forward

As we conclude this chapter, it's vital to acknowledge that the journey ahead may not always be straightforward. The human brain is a marvel of complexity and resilience, and our understanding of it continues to evolve. Therefore, before delving further into the intricacies of this profound subject, it's essential to approach the forthcoming information with an open mind and a critical eye. Every individual's brain health journey is unique, shaped by a myriad of factors, including genetics, environment, lifestyle, and unforeseen events. While this book strives to provide valuable insights and guidance, it's crucial to remember that no single source can encapsulate the full spectrum of experiences related to brain health. Hence, I encourage you, the reader, to embrace this information as a stepping stone rather than a definitive answer. At the heart of this book lies a sincere desire to empower and inform, but it's important to emphasize the significance of seeking personalized, professional advice when navigating matters pertaining to brain health. Each person's circumstances warrant tailored approaches, and the expertise of healthcare professionals can offer invaluable support and direction in addressing specific concerns or conditions. As we embark on the subsequent chapters, let's maintain an appreciative and discerning mindset. While the content presented here aims to enrich your understanding, always remember that self-care and well-being extend beyond knowledge alone. In intertwining the latest scientific findings with compassionate human experiences, we aspire to foster an environment of empathy and shared learning. Before we venture forth, take a moment to reflect on your personal intentions for engaging with this material. Whether you seek practical strategies, scientific insights, or simply a deeper empathetic connection with the concept of brain health, each objective is equally valid and worthy. Embrace the upcoming chapters as opportunities for growth, self-discovery, and a strengthened commitment to holistic well-being. In the spirit of continual learning, let's approach the ensuing content with humility, curiosity, and an unwavering dedication to promoting mental health and cognitive vitality. May these final words serve as a gentle reminder to proceed with both confidence and reverence, honoring the intricate tapestry of the human brain while recognizing the boundless possibilities for nurturing its well-being.

Conclusion

Reflection on Key Insights

Understanding the brain is fundamental to appreciating its complexities. As we reflect on the wealth of knowledge presented in this book, it is clear that the intricate world within our minds holds immeasurable significance. From unraveling the anatomy of the brain to exploring the intricate network of neurons, every revelation has opened doors to a deeper collective understanding. We have delved into the role of vitamins and nutrients, recognizing the vital support they offer for optimal brain function. The profound impact of exercise and physical activity on our mental well-being has become evident, highlighting the interconnectedness of body and mind. Our exploration of nutrition and diet has unearthed the profound influence that dietary choices wield over cognitive health. Through the exploration of medical insights and treatments, we have gained insight into the remarkable progress being made in the field of neurological care. Recent scientific studies have offered fresh perspectives, igniting hope and inspiring further inquiry into the enigmatic domain of the brain. Real-life case studies and personal stories have humanized the complex subject matter, resonating with readers on a deeply personal level. Practical tips for everyday care have empowered us to make tangible changes in our daily lives, nurturing our brain's well-being. While our understanding may be vast, it is essential to acknowledge the challenges and limitations that still exist in our knowledge of the brain. It is through acknowledging these gaps that we can pave the way for future discoveries and breakthroughs. The power of community and support has underscored the importance of standing together in our quest for brain health. Looking ahead, we see a path illuminated by possibilities and potential. As we conclude this journey, we express gratitude for the opportunity to delve into the intricacies of the brain, cultivating a deeper connection with our own cognition. Our pursuit of knowledge and well-being is an ongoing endeavor, and may we carry the torch of curiosity and understanding forward, embracing the lifelong exploration of the wondrous terrain within our minds.

Collective Understanding

As we conclude this journey through the complexities of the brain, it becomes increasingly evident that knowledge alone is not enough; it is our collective understanding that has the power to effect real, tangible change in our lives and the lives of those around us. Our individual experiences, discoveries, and learnings, when combined with those of others, form a rich tapestry of insight and understanding. It is through sharing and listening to these diverse perspectives that we cultivate a true collective understanding of the intricate workings of the brain and its impact on our overall well-being. Our collective understanding extends beyond mere academic or medical knowledge; it encompasses the deeply personal stories of individuals who have bravely navigated their own paths through challenges related to brain health. These stories serve as a reminder that our shared experiences bind us together, creating a powerful network of empathy and support. In this interconnected web of human experiences, we find solace, motivation, and inspiration to strive for better brain health for ourselves and for those we care about. It is through our collective understanding that we come to appreciate the significance of fostering a culture of openness, acceptance, and inclusivity. Every voice adds value to this discourse, and every unique perspective contributes to a more comprehensive understanding of the intricacies of the brain. Perhaps most importantly, our collective understanding allows us to advocate for positive changes in our communities, driving awareness and support for mental health resources, research initiatives, and accessible care. This understanding also compels us to recognize and address the existing stigma surrounding brain-related conditions, opening up discussions that shatter misconceptions and lead to compassionate action. Together, we can work towards establishing environments where individuals feel safe to seek help and where their concerns are met with understanding, respect, and genuine support. In conclusion, our collective understanding serves as an invaluable foundation upon which we can build a brighter, healthier future for all. Through this shared comprehension, we foster strength, resilience, and compassion, propelling us towards a world where the complexities of the brain are met with empathy and understanding.

Realizing Change Through Knowledge

Understanding the intricate workings of the brain leads to the empowering realization that change is within our grasp. Armed with knowledge about the brain's remarkable adaptability and response to various stimuli, individuals are equipped to pursue positive transformations in their lives. By comprehending the impact of environment, lifestyle, and mental engagement on brain health, we unveil a path towards meaningful and lasting change. This journey isn't just about altering habits; it's about fostering a deep understanding of how our choices shape our brain's function and structure. As the convergence of neuroscience and psychology continues to shed light on the incredible plasticity of the brain, we are presented with an array of opportunities to actively influence our cognitive well-being through education, awareness, and intentional actions. The notion of realizing change through knowledge is not a lofty ideal but a tangible reality supported by scientific evidence and personal experiences. With this understanding, individuals can engage in purposeful endeavors that support cognitive growth and resilience. Furthermore, by recognizing the interconnected nature of the mind and body, individuals can embrace holistic approaches to well-being, wherein they honor not only their brain's vitality but also their overall health. This profound recognition fosters a sense of agency and responsibility, inspiring individuals to make informed choices that encompass physical, emotional, and cognitive dimensions. Realizing change through knowledge evokes a profound shift in perspective, propelling individuals towards a proactive stance in optimizing their brain health and overall wellness. It prompts a departure from passive acceptance of circumstances to an active pursuit of flourishing. This paradigm acknowledges the potential for transformative progress and celebrates the capacity of each individual to contribute to their own well-being. Ultimately, as we internalize the significance of knowledge in steering positive change, we open ourselves to a world of possibilities where personal growth, resilience, and fulfillment thrive.

The Journey to Better Health

Achieving better health is not merely a destination; rather, it's an on-going journey requiring dedication, perseverance, and continual learning. As we pave our paths towards improved well-being, it's important to recognize that the process is far from linear. It involves embracing various aspects of wellness, which encompass physical, mental, and emotional dimensions. This journey begins with self-awareness, understanding our bodies' needs, limitations, and unique requirements. Through this awareness, we can cultivate healthier habits, including balanced nutrition, regular exercise, and mindful practices that nourish both body and mind. Moreover, as we progress, it becomes evident that the journey to better health doesn't occur in isolation. It intertwines with our relationships, environment, and community. Engaging and seeking support from like-minded individuals can significantly impact our overall well-being, providing accountability, encouragement, and shared experiences. The journey also entails confronting and overcoming obstacles, setbacks, and moments of doubt. It's about resilience and adaptability, understanding that setbacks are part of growth, and using them as opportunities for reflection and reevaluation. Along this path, there will be periods of immense progress, coupled with plateau phases and even temporary regression. Embracing the entire spectrum of this journey equips us with resilience, fostering the ability to navigate life's ebbs and flows while maintaining a steadfast commitment to our health. This pursuit holds the potential to elevate our lives in profound ways, enhancing our vitality, energy, and overall outlook. The journey to better health transcends mere physical changes; it encompasses a holistic transformation, enriching our daily experiences and nurturing a sustainable, thriving lifestyle. Embracing this journey requires consistent dedication, yet the rewards extend beyond individual benefit. By prioritizing our health, we become better equipped to fulfill our duties, engage with our loved ones, and contribute positively to our communities. It's a journey that propels us towards becoming the best versions of ourselves, instilling a sense of purpose, fulfillment, and resilience. As we chart this course toward better health, we embark on a transformative odyssey that cultivates lasting, meaningful change.

Embracing Lifelong Learning

Lifelong learning is a fundamental aspect of our human experience, and it holds immense significance in the context of understanding the complexities of brain health. The concept of embracing lifelong learning goes beyond mere accumulation of knowledge; it encompasses a mindset that fosters intellectual curiosity, open-mindedness, and a continuous thirst for new information and experiences. As we navigate through the various stages of life, it becomes increasingly clear that remaining receptive to learning opportunities contributes significantly to our overall well-being. Embracing lifelong learning can enrich our lives in profound ways, serving as a catalyst for personal growth and development. One of the most beautiful aspects of embracing lifelong learning is the innate sense of wonder and discovery that it evokes. It encourages us to approach the world with fresh eyes, allowing us to find joy and fascination in the simplest of things. This active engagement with the world around us stimulates our cognitive functions, igniting the creative spark within us and nurturing a sense of fulfillment. Whether it's delving into a new subject, exploring different cultures, or acquiring practical skills, the pursuit of knowledge empowers us to expand our perspectives and cultivate a deeper understanding of the world we inhabit. Moreover, embracing lifelong learning has a remarkable impact on our mental acuity and resilience. Research has shown that continued intellectual stimulation is linked to enhanced cognitive function and a reduced risk of cognitive decline as we age. By actively seeking out new challenges and learning experiences, we exercise our brains, fortifying neural pathways and cognitive reserves. This proactive approach to mental agility equips us with the cognitive resources needed to adapt to changing circumstances and maintain a resilient mind, bolstering our capacity to overcome obstacles and thrive in the face of adversity. On a broader societal level, embracing lifelong learning promotes a culture of empathy, understanding, and inclusivity. It fosters an environment where diverse perspectives are celebrated, and individuals are encouraged to engage in meaningful dialogue and exchange of ideas. This inclusive approach not only broadens our horizons but also cultivates a deep sense of empathy and interconnectedness with others. Moreover, by staying informed about emerging research and developments in the field of brain health, we can actively contribute to the dissemination of knowledge and advocate for equitable access to resources and support for all members of society. In essence, embracing lifelong learning is a transformative and empowering journey that transcends age, background, and circumstance. It enables us to lead fulfilling lives marked by intellectual vitality, resilience, and a profound connection to the world around us. By embracing the ethos of lifelong learning, we not only enrich our own lives but also contribute to the collective growth and well-being of our communities. As we continue to explore the depths of knowledge and experience, let us embrace the boundless potential that lifelong learning offers and celebrate the wondrous journey of discovery and self-discovery.

Encouragement for Continued Exploration

In our journey to understanding the complexities of the brain, the pursuit of knowledge is an ongoing and deeply rewarding endeavor.

As we continue to navigate the vast landscape of neuroscience, let us embrace the spirit of curiosity and intellectual exploration. Each new discovery and insight serves to enrich our understanding and appreciation of this remarkable organ. Through a commitment to lifelong learning, we empower ourselves to seek out novel perspectives and innovative approaches. It is through this continuous exploration that we cultivate a profound sense of intellectual fulfillment and personal growth. Furthermore, embracing continued exploration allows us to remain adaptable in the face of evolving scientific advancements. The field of neuroscience is constantly evolving, with new research shedding light on previously uncharted territories. By acknowledging the dynamic nature of this discipline, we position ourselves to engage with emerging concepts and breakthroughs. In doing so, we foster a mindset of adaptability and open-mindedness, enabling us to integrate new knowledge into our existing framework of understanding. This willingness to venture into uncharted intellectual territory not only expands our individual horizons but also contributes to the collective progression of neurological science. Moreover, the encouragement for continued exploration extends beyond personal enrichment; it serves as a catalyst for innovation and progress within the broader scientific community. As we delve deeper into the intricacies of the brain, our collective efforts contribute to a comprehensive tapestry of insights that propel the field forward. This collaborative spirit of exploration fuels a climate of creativity and discovery, where diverse perspectives converge to unravel the mysteries of the mind. By actively participating in this expansive discourse, we contribute to a legacy of knowledge that transcends individual contributions, leaving an indelible mark on the landscape of neurological research. Ultimately, the journey of continued exploration is characterized by its transformative power. It offers us the opportunity to transcend preconceived boundaries, transcend preconceived boundaries, challenging us to think critically and expansively.

Embracing the inherent uncertainties of exploration fosters resilience and fortitude, equipping us with the courage to confront the unknown. This bold pursuit of knowledge fuels our intellectual passion and bolsters our capacity to effect meaningful change in the realm of neuroscience and beyond. Therefore, let us heed the call to embrace continued exploration, recognizing it as both a personal and collective undertaking that enriches our lives and shapes the future of neurological understanding.

Acknowledging Challenges and Limitations

As we come to the conclusion of this journey through the complexities of the human brain, it's important to take a moment to acknowledge the challenges and limitations that we may encounter along the way. Despite our best efforts and intentions, there are bound to be obstacles that we must confront in our quest for understanding and nurturing the brain. One of the fundamental challenges is the ever-evolving nature of scientific knowledge. The field of neuroscience is continuously expanding, with new discoveries and breakthroughs reshaping our understanding of the brain. While this progress is incredibly exciting, it also means that we must stay adaptable and open-minded, ready to revise our perspectives in the face of emerging information. Additionally, we must recognize the limitations of our current scientific and medical capabilities. There are still numerous aspects of the brain that remain enigmatic, and conditions such as neurodegenerative disorders present profound challenges in terms of treatment and management. It's crucial to approach these limitations with humility and a commitment to persistent inquiry and innovation. Beyond the realm of science, societal attitudes and stigmas surrounding mental health constitute another formidable obstacle. Despite significant strides in advocacy and awareness, there persists a pervasive misunderstanding and discrimination against individuals dealing with neurological and psychological conditions. Addressing these deep-seated societal challenges demands sustained effort and compassion from all members of our global community. Moreover, on an individual level, we must confront the personal barriers that may impede our pursuit of brain health and well-being. Whether it's overcoming ingrained habits, managing time constraints, or navigating complex healthcare systems, each of us faces unique hurdles that call for resilience and perseverance. In acknowledging these challenges and limitations, we do not succumb to pessimism. Instead, we fortify ourselves with the awareness that progress is often born out of adversity. By embracing these difficulties with courage and determination, we can channel our collective energies towards fostering a deeper understanding of the brain and cultivating a more supportive and empathetic environment for all those impacted by neurological conditions. This acknowledgment serves as a reminder that our journey towards enhancing brain health is an ongoing, dynamic process—one that requires both fortitude in the face of challenges and a steadfast commitment to driving positive change.

The Power of Community and Support

In our journey to understand the complexities of the human brain and how it impacts our overall well-being, we must recognize the immense power of community and support. It is through the interconnectedness of individuals that we find strength, empathy, and transformative change. The power of community lies in its ability to nurture and uplift, offering a sense of belonging and understanding. When faced with the challenges of nurturing a healthy mind and body, the support of a like-minded community can be the cornerstone of resilience. Whether it's the camaraderie found in a local wellness group, the unwavering encouragement from friends and family, or the compassion extended by online networks, the impact of community support cannot be understated. At times, the path to better health may seem daunting, but together, as a community, we can celebrate victories, share knowledge, and provide solace during moments of struggle. This collective strength amplifies the potential for positive change and fosters an environment where individuals feel empowered to prioritize their well-being. Moreover, the exchange of experiences within a supportive community allows for the validation of individual journeys and fosters a spirit of inclusivity. As we recognize the unique challenges each person faces, a community becomes a source of comfort, guidance, and motivation. It is within this web of interconnectedness that stories are shared, learning is facilitated, and hope is ignited. The significance of community and support extends beyond personal benefit; it permeates societal structures and redefines the way we approach holistic health. By fostering a culture of understanding and caring, communities become a force for positive influence, shaping environments that prioritize mental and physical well-being. As we collectively navigate the complexities of life, the bonds formed within a compassionate community serve as anchors of stability and sources of inspiration. Let us not underestimate the transformative power of coming together, for it is within the embrace of a supportive community that we find the courage to embark on the path toward enhanced well-being.

Looking Forward: The Path Ahead

As we conclude this insightful journey into the complexities and wonders of the human brain, it is essential to look forward and acknowledge the paths that lie ahead. The knowledge and understanding gained from exploring the intricate workings of the brain have opened doors to a new level of awareness and potential for growth. It is imperative to recognize that this newfound awareness is not the end, but rather the beginning of a continuous journey towards better cognitive health and overall well-being. Looking ahead, it becomes evident that the path to optimal brain health is paved with ongoing learning, empowerment, and proactive involvement. Embracing the path ahead involves a commitment to further educate ourselves, integrate healthy practices into our daily lives, and advocate for the importance of mental wellness within our communities and society as a whole. With the overarching goal of fostering a culture of brain health and resilience, the path ahead also entails the recognition of individual strengths and the collective power of a supportive community. Engaging in open dialogues, sharing experiences, and offering support to those in need form the core of building a network that fosters understanding, empathy, and solidarity. Together, we can pave the way for a more inclusive, compassionate, and supportive environment for everyone on their journey to improved brain health. Moreover, the path ahead must navigate through the ever-evolving landscape of scientific advancements, medical breakthroughs, and innovative technologies. With these tools at our disposal, there is great potential to unlock new possibilities for enhancing brain function, treating neurological conditions, and promoting mental resilience. It is crucial to remain informed about these advancements and actively participate in discussions that shape the future of brain health research and care. Looking forward also necessitates recognizing the importance of self-care and making conscious choices that prioritize mental and physical well-being. By incorporating mindfulness practices, maintaining a balanced diet, engaging in regular exercise, and seeking moments of rejuvenation, we can embark on a path that nurtures the mind, body, and spirit. Furthermore, as we set our sights on the road ahead, it is crucial to embrace resilience and adaptability in the face of challenges. Recognizing that setbacks and obstacles may arise on this journey, we can cultivate the strength to persevere and find creative solutions to overcome adversity. This resilience empowers us to continuously evolve and thrive amidst the dynamic nature of life. In essence, the path ahead calls for a deepened sense of responsibility, compassion, and dedication to our own well-being and that of others. By collectively looking forward with optimism, determination, and an unwavering commitment to nurturing the brain's potential, we can pave a transformative path that leads to enhanced cognitive health, enriched lives, and a more vibrant future for generations to come.

Parting Thoughts and Expressing Gratitude

In concluding this insightful journey through the complexities of the brain, it's essential to express sincere gratitude to everyone who has contributed to the creation of this book. As we reflect on the wealth of knowledge we've uncovered, there is an overwhelming sense of appreciation for the collective effort that went into bringing this work to fruition. It's with heartfelt thanks that we acknowledge the researchers, medical professionals, and individuals who shared their personal experiences and stories, enriching the fabric of this narrative. Gratitude extends beyond those directly involved in the creation of this book. We appreciate every reader who has embarked on this exploration of the human brain. Your engagement and curiosity have been the driving force behind our commitment to providing valuable insights and practical guidance for enhancing brain health and well-being. The support and encouragement from family, friends, and mentors have been invaluable throughout this endeavor. Their unwavering belief in the importance of advocating for brain health has inspired us to delve deeper into this subject, seeking a comprehensive understanding that we could share with you, the reader. For their patience, understanding, and unwavering support, we extend our deepest gratitude. As we part ways at the conclusion of this book, it's important to carry forward the enthusiasm and commitment to preserving and promoting brain health. Our gratitude evolves into a call to action, a reminder that the knowledge gained should be applied in our daily lives, shared with others, and continued to be explored and expanded upon. Let's embark on the future with the knowledge that a community dedicated to brain health is a powerful force for positive change. In parting, know that your interest in the well-being of the brain leaves an indelible mark on the collective efforts to advance research, understanding, and care. Your role in fostering awareness and championing the cause of brain health is both appreciated and essential. With deep gratitude and a hopeful outlook, we bid you farewell, carrying the bond of shared knowledge and inspiring potential. Thank you for joining us on this enlightening journey.

Did you love *Understanding The Body The Brain*? Then you should read *Mind Over Memory Boosting Cognitive Function After 60*[1] by Robert Jakobsen!

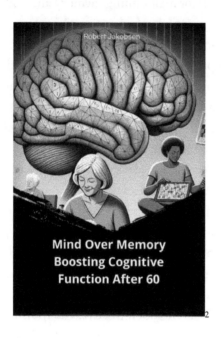
[2]

Mind Over Memory: Boosting Cognitive Function After 60 is an essential guide for anyone looking to maintain and improve their memory and cognitive abilities as they age. In a world where aging is often associated with decline, this book offers a refreshing and empowering perspective on how to keep your brain sharp and resilient well into your golden years.

Drawing on the latest scientific research and practical strategies, Mind Over Memory delves into the factors that influence cognitive health. From understanding how memory works to recognizing the

1. https://books2read.com/u/38lJ8w

2. https://books2read.com/u/38lJ8w

difference between normal age-related changes and signs of cognitive decline, this book is designed to provide actionable insights for readers.

Inside, you'll explore:

The importance of maintaining memory and cognitive function as you age

How lifestyle choices like physical exercise, diet, and social engagement can protect and even enhance brain health

Techniques and exercises designed to keep your mind sharp and boost memory retention

How stress, mental health, and sleep impact cognitive function and what you can do to improve them

The link between lifelong learning, hobbies, and neuroplasticity — the brain's ability to grow and adapt

Whether you're experiencing mild forgetfulness or are simply looking for ways to stay mentally agile, this book provides a wealth of information and practical advice to help you embrace aging with a healthy mind. It's time to defy the stereotypes of aging and reclaim your mental clarity, independence, and vitality.

With Mind Over Memory, discover the tools you need to unlock your brain's potential and live a more vibrant, fulfilling life—no matter your age.

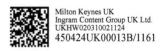

Milton Keynes UK
Ingram Content Group UK Ltd.
UKHW020310021124
450424UK00013B/1161

9 798227 546937